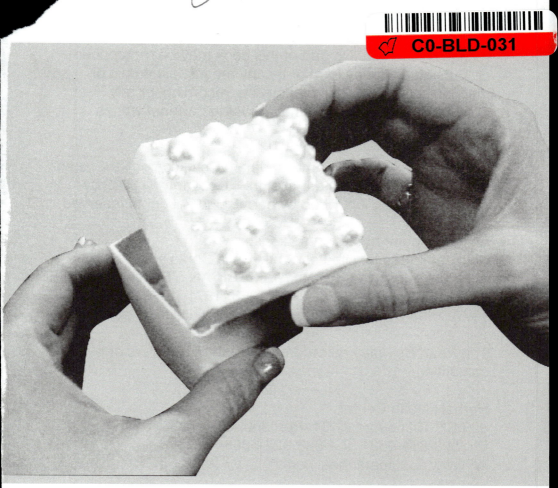

The Pearl Box

Breaking the bondage of disease through Biblical tools
for physical, mental, emotional, and spiritual health.

SYLVIA ROGERS

The Pearl Box may be ordered through booksellers or by contacting:

Herbal Health Center
829 SE 182nd Ave # 101, Portland, OR 97233, USA
Ph: 503-661-0631 or 1-888-327-5666
W: www.equippedtoheal.com

$15.95 each.
Volume discounts may apply.
Please E-mail your testimonies!

ISBN: 978-1-4675-6184-6

Design by **Bethany Talbert**
Printed in India by **devtechprinters.com**

Disclaimer

The publisher, author, distributors, and any sellers of this book present this information for educational purposes alone. None of its contents are intended to diagnose or prescribe for any medical or psychological conditions. The author, publisher, and sellers do not intend any of this information to claim to prevent, treat, mitigate, or cure any disease, disorder, or condition. This book is not intended to replace one's doctor or qualified health practitioner. This book is a sharing of knowledge and experience only. Testimonials are shared, but should not be construed as results that others will experience as a certainty. Everyone is unique in their own journey of spiritual healing and what they experience. Everything within this publication is for the purpose of aligning ourselves with our Creator's design for optimal spiritual health on every level of our being. This author believes all true healing is spiritual healing through alignment to our Creator's intents and purposes for us. This entire book is spiritually based and any cure experienced is attributed to the work of God made manifest through our obedience to His wonderful spiritual health principles. Any reference to products or healing tools are for general teaching purposes for further investigation by readers as they design their own personal health journey. All readers are encouraged to make their own personal health care decisions based upon their own study ad partnership with their health professionals. You alone, as the reader, are responsible for any and all you choose to do regarding anything you read and implement within this publication.

Important: I have had a few clients give feedback that they experienced some dizziness after beginning some of the spiritual exercises within. Therefore, please use caution if driving or in any potentially unsafe scenario should any similar experiences occur. These exercises may have a powerful potential to assist the body in toxin release and clearance. Start slowly to begin and always listen to your body's feedback.

"Thank you, Sylvia, for *The Pearl Box*. My medical staff are able to help many people heal emotionally by directing them to your book and letting God do all the rest. We are having customers send folks in that have never been in our facility just to get *The Pearl Box*! My staff and I have all had some unexpected releases by reading and helping others speak out the affirmations in your book. I hear nothing but positive feed back from my clients who have read its many "pearls." I also really appreciate the Scripture references and that they are written out for us to read."

- Kelly Sandelius, ND
Certified Naturopathic Doctor
Certified Herbalist
Certified Natural Health Professional
www.healthybasicsinc.com

CONTENTS

Acknowledgements   ix

The Pearl Box   x

Author's Note   xii

Introduction   1

Part One Pearls of Physical Health   13

Part Two Pearls of Mental Health   57

Part Three Pearls of Emotional Health   84

Part Four Pearls of Spiritual Health   144

Part Five Using Your Pearls   158

Appendix I The Salvation Blueprint   165

Appendix II Tools for Cleansing   170

Appendix III Renew Your Mind, Transform Your Body   173

Appendix IV Sample Prayers for Trauma & Healing   186

Appendix V Godly Solutions for Healthy Sleep   190

Appendix VI Ellie's Prayer for the Spine   193

Appendix VII Prayers for Conception & Pregnancy   196

Appendix VIII Total Forgiveness   199

Appendix IX Cleansing Your Home   200

Appendix X Testimonies   201

Appendix XI The Teacup Story   206

Acknowledgements

I am very grateful for the initial encouragement and inspiration of my family, my "Pearlbox Ladies," and my friend, Lynn, who inspired the initial "aha" moment in the development of this study.

I am especially grateful to our great God, Jehovah Rapha, who heals body, mind, emotions, and spirit. He has through all the years inspired me with His great Words containing these precious pearls.

I dedicate this book to my readers in their pursuit of optimal health and well-being. God bless your journey!

The Pearl Box

It sat in my home, hidden for years
while life went on with laughter and tears.
I studied God's Word, handed down through the ages,
Unaware priceless pearls still hid in its pages.

I pondered the world, in illness and pain,
And the people in church, who suffered the same.
So I focused on wellness for my life and family,
Embracing a natural health mentality

I opened an herb store, using my talents
To help my family and hundreds of clients.
But no matter my efforts to find what was best,
Something key was missing in my wellness quest.

One day my eyes opened in a miraculous way.
A Christian speaker proclaimed, "God still heals today!"
Look for the pearls encased in the large,
Yearning for discovery and free of charge.

"How can this be?" I asked, for I'd heard many a prayer,
That seemed to bypass God and fall into thin air.
You see, Satan deceives, he loves to tell lies:
"There's little you can do. God has closed His eyes!"

But we each have a box, into which pearls may go,
From whose gleaming clusters healing powers flow.

By Christ's stripes, we have been healed—past tense!
Let's confidently claim this, then use common sense.

Look again and see, broaden your sight—
Onto what are you holding, hidden from light?
Many of your pains have been buried for years;
Often overflowing with anger and tears.

We've bottled old sorrows, bitterness, and blame,
Plus many other things we prefer not to name--
And remaining in mire, through struggles so rife
We miss God's blessings and a chance at new life.

But we serve a Holy God who yearns to bless us so.
In Him, we are forgiven, but these strongholds must go.
"Get out, negative thinking, buried anger, and strife!"
It's time to search our souls and expel these outright.

Evict aloud - old heartbreak, worry, shame…,
"Go out from my being, in Jesus' holy name!"
There's some repentance to do and He is faithful to forgive,
Become God's great masterpiece--stand up and live!

Now gather your pearls, so beautiful and bright--
And lay claim to their healing against all darkness in your life.

--Sylvia Rogers

Author's Note

I believe all true healing is under the umbrella of spiritual healing; a realigning of our entire being with the divine precepts of God, our Creator. For years, I have believed that God wants better for us than we can envision. However, we all see people who frequently voice doubt in divine provision, especially for their physical healing, with the exception of the strength to simply endure it.

Have you ever implored God, "Where are Your answers to cancer, diabetes, arthritis, and heart disease?" or, "How do I cope with the anger, sorrow, and worry that torment me? What about my negative thinking patterns? I say things that I hate saying and do things that I hate doing. God help me!"

If God seems silent, we often transfer these burdens to our doctors, who struggle mightily to find a scientific cure, but who often resort to using suppressive medications as well as surgeries as coping tools.

If you have been down this path, you are not alone. We all want answers and in the despair of not getting them, many of us repeatedly ask God for miraculous healing. Let me ask you this: "Why do we not also ask God to mow our lawns, fill our cars with gas, or cook our meals?" This seems a bit silly because we have been given the obvious tools to do these ourselves. But what about the tools for our best health? Is it possible that God has already given these to us also?

All Scripture is given by inspiration of God, and is profitable for doctrine, for reproof, for correction, for instruction in righteousness, that the man of God maybe complete, thoroughly equipped for every good work (2 Tim 3:16-17).

This Scripture does not say *partially equipped* but *thoroughly equipped* for EVERY good work!

Is ridding ourselves of any personal health challenge a good work? What if God's tools are right in front of us and we are just not seeing them? Society and its teachings have a profound effect on how we *see.* Even our religious teachers are influenced in their healing and health advice by the current Western medical model of health.

Through the years, I have investigated traditional (Western) medicine, alternative medicine, the writings and works of Christian healers Henry Wright, Keith Moore, Caroline Leaf, and others, as well as observed multiple client data through biofeedback and analysis. With the addition of much prayer and meditation on God's Word, I am convinced that God has already provided the majority of our healing through the power present in His living pearls of wisdom and health contained within the Bible.

However, the overall mentality of today's society encourages us to look to science for answers. Yes, we may find ways to help ourselves, but it often comes with a price as we struggle to make the best choices with the knowledge base we have.

I do not believe God faults us for this, but I believe He has a better and more excellent way.

But earnestly desire the best gifts. And yet I show you a more excellent way (1 Cor 12:31).

God has our best at heart and desires to give us excellence in all things. Our challenge is in recognizing the gifts that He has given.

Over two thousand years ago, a bold woman with her finances and health options exhausted, put her faith into action by touching the hem of Christ's garment, thereby accessing the flow of His healing power:

> *And, behold, a woman, which was diseased with an issue of blood twelve years, came behind him, and touched the hem of his garment: for she said within herself, If I may but touch his garment, I shall be whole. But Jesus turned him about, and when he saw her, he said, Daughter, be of good comfort; thy faith hath made thee whole. And the woman was made whole from that hour (Matt 9:20-22).*

> *And when the men of that place had knowledge of him, they sent out into all that country roundabout, and brought unto him all that were diseased; and besought him that they might only touch the hem of his garment: and as many as touched were made perfectly whole (Matt 14:35-36).*

I believe we are generously afforded a similar opportunity. In faith, expecting results, we can grab hold of the Christ, who is accessible to all of us as the powerful Word of God.

> *And the Word became flesh and dwelt among us, and we beheld His glory, the glory as of the only begotten of the Father, full of grace and truth (John 1:14-15).*

In laying claim to God's Words—infused with the power of His Holy Spirit--and proclaiming them over our challenges, we are, in essence, taking hold of "the hem" and allowing the healing power of Christ to become active in all aspects of our lives and health.

Within this study, we will obtain biblical tools to cast off the habits and patterns that may bind us to disease. With the cultivation of our faith, let us not simply read God's Word, but lay verbal claim regularly to His excellent pearls of power, might, and healing that He has already given us (past tense) through His Son's sacrifice, to live the abundant life of health that He intended. Here is a powerful healing promise that we can verbally personalize and claim frequently (note the condition):

who Himself bore our sins in His own body on the tree, that we, having died to sins, might live for righteousness— by whose stripes you were healed (1 Peter 2:24).

By Christ's stripes I have been healed (past tense)! The tools are here, now. If you have died to sin (see Appendix 1), claim this Scripture with conviction.

When accessing God's beautiful healing pearls, we rejoice that from Christ's amazing sacrifice, death, burial, and resurrection, the kingdom of heaven, the finest pearl of all, has been made available. It is the Father's most precious gift to us and the means to eternal life with Him. Perfect health is the effortless norm in heaven.

Again, the kingdom of heaven is like a merchant seeking beautiful pearls, who, when he had found one pearl of great price, went and sold all that he had and bought it (Matt 13:45-46).

Within this beautiful offering, there is an array of beautiful, priceless, and unique smaller pearls to discover.

Activating them in our lives is the key.

This next principle is extremely important. As we read the many Scriptures pertaining to our health, let us claim them aloud. *Speaking* God's Word is a powerful activator of its power.

When my clients speak Scriptures and spiritual principles during biofeedback, dramatic stress-reducing physical and emotional shifts are recorded. Stress patterns come in all forms and are taught to be the root of at least 80% of our illnesses. Life and death truly reside in the power of the tongue, as the Bible teaches. As we speak God's Word over our lives, our bodies, minds, and emotions (all our spiritual energies within) are free to move into harmonious alignment, as God intended.

In this study, you will be challenged to release negative, health-damaging practices and replace their vacancies with sound beliefs and healthy habits, not once but many times, until they become memorized and engrafted into your being.

God's power is unleashed through the vehicle of His Word and we are created in His image. When we speak His words and principles over ourselves, we come into contact with the amazing power of God and change begins to happen!

Introduction

I must begin by expressing gratitude to my mother for her strong foundational influence on this journey of discovery. She was a strong woman who loved the Lord and stood up for what she believed.

I remember the day when she took my gentle, sweet grandfather, James, to the doctor. He lived with us and was taking more and more to his bed from stiffness and soreness in his muscles and joints. Two specialists diagnosed a "muscular form of arthritis" and offered little hope-- "after all, he's over 85 years old."

I was only nine or ten years old at that time, but I remember my mother rejecting that bleak diagnosis and actively looking into the natural health field for hopeful solutions. We both began attending yearly National Health Federation conventions featuring expert speakers who shared a wealth of 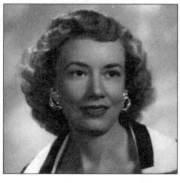 information on natural health topics. We enjoyed many impassioned lectures on healing the body naturally taught by devoted health pioneers and authors, such as expert nutritionist Dr. Bernard Jensen, Master Herbalist Dr. John Christopher, and author, lecturer Betty Lee Morales. They and others were forging an uphill battle in the age of "Better Living through Chemistry."

In America, pharmaceuticals were exploding in popularity. Nevertheless, my mother and I continued to enjoy attending these conventions, and weekly visits to the health-food store became routine.

I still have memories of her discussions with the store's owner, Tom. She was intent on a mission to see just what her healthy options were outside of the limited nutritional knowledge within the medical realm.

My mother came home armed with organic foods, a vegetable juicer, carrots, beets, apples, vitamins, minerals, and plenty of determination. With perseverance, Grandpa not only got out of bed, he stayed out! He puttered around, washed the dishes, worked in the yard, and hacked out some old tree stumps. In his nineties, he jetted to Spain and Hawaii. His 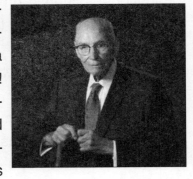 mind was always as sharp as a tack, and he could tell you the date of any event upon which he related. I saw him as a walking encyclopedia.

My grandpa proclaimed regularly that he desired to live to be 100 years old. True to what he spoke, he enjoyed his 100th birthday. A few days later, he felt a chill enter his body and five days after that, he peacefully passed away.

As I entered my teen years, my interest in health continued to grow. I enrolled in a four-year nursing program at the University of Portland and graduated with honors.

I enjoyed my studies, but I observed many patients whom I believed could have better results with the addition of natural healing tools. I pursued specialized studies in nutrition for the following year where I learned to design nutritional programs for various organs and systems of the body. I also took a local class entitled *Herbs for Health*. I had a strong desire to be knowledge-able and responsible for my family's well-being. Meanwhile, I continued working in nursing but began teaching principles of cleansing, healthy eating, and herbal medicine on the side.

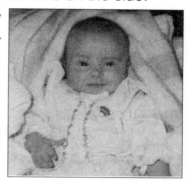

I was continually amazed at my clients' results and testimonies. A year later, I gave birth to my first child. I used herbs and vitamins before and during my pregnancy. With a midwife's assistance, I had a four-hour labor and a home birth using no medication.

My second birth, though natural, took place in a hospital as my daughter was breech. Again, us-ing herbal formulas, my labor lasted only four hours. My doctor proclaimed it to be "the easiest breech delivery" he had seen "in 20 years!"

My last child, an easy birth at home, was also born naturally without medications.

My children were raised happy and healthy in a positive home environment using only natural remedies with the excep-tion of dental treatments, setting a broken bone, and receiving a few stitches.

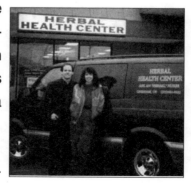

As the use of natural medicine became routine in our lives, my hus-band and I opened The Herbal Health Center storefront to share with others what we had learned and to provide a source of quality herbs, vitamins, supplements, and essential oils.

We carefully chose Nature's Sunshine Products, a line of approximately 600 nutritional supplements due to their quality, company integrity, and cutting-edge educational programs.

Now, more than 25 years later, I can no longer count the testimonies of satisfied clients who claimed new leases on life using natural approaches. I could not ask for a better career, and often muse about how I have come to this point from my initial journey in nursing school. I am so grateful to the Lord for having taken my quest for the truths of health and fulfilling it far better than I could have ever envisioned.

In the spring of 2008, a pivotal event occurred while using biofeedback with a client on a software program that graphs both emotional and physical stress patterns. The program indicated excess stress in her emotional graph. She felt that this had its roots in a serious office rift she had with a coworker that involved anger and residues of unforgiveness.

"I am not taking those frogs home with me!" she proclaimed in my office before spontaneously praying aloud, denouncing and releasing the emotional stress patterns, one by one, and giving them to the Lord. Like an amazing drama unfolding before my eyes, I saw the peaked portions on the graph revert back into the normal range from her impassioned words! Impressive! It definitely got my attention.

Now, after countless experiments with consenting clients, I have seen similar results each time they used verbal proclamations, commands, and prayers, reflected not just on the emotional graph, but also on the screens showing physical stress. To my delight, when clients employed these healing tools, the reliance on supplements for detoxification decreased. Clients shared that many of their symptoms such as aches, pains, and inflammation began to alleviate on their own.

These fascinating observations regarding the mind-body-emotional-spiritual connections are not really new. The Bible, written thousands of years ago, speaks of it, and science continues to add its support.

What follows is an adventure of discovery into God's multi-faceted approach to health and what we may learn and act upon to receive His blessings in these areas from the amazing pearls He has provided.

Standing at the Crossroads

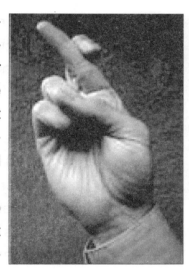

If you have been perceiving disease as a bad lottery ticket, crossing your fingers and hoping that your number does not pop up, then maybe it is time to take a new look at what you believe. Your current frame of reference may not reflect God's eternal truths.

Let us be truth seekers--free to change our minds and habits in pursuit of God's standards for our lives. Believe that your life is going to change!

Jesus said to him, "If you can believe, all things are possible to him who believes" (Mark 9:23).

Reading this book through several times will yield the best results. Each time, different portions will speak louder than others as you grow. This journey requires time, change, and regular homework. It also means peering (not wallowing) into the abyss of your various strongholds to locate the old dirt and cobwebs that need sweeping away.

We will also take a look at imprinted character and emotional patterns that may have come from ancesteral connections, as these may be playing a part in holding your health in bondage.

Many blessings will result from taking these first steps, coupled with the tears of emotional release, vulnerability to God's Word, newly-set goals, and victories over the inevitable attacks by the dark forces of this world that want us to stay ill, discontent, and miserable like they are. The greatest blessing of all will be increased faith in the loving provision of our Lord, recognizing that our lives are a wonderful masterpiece in progress as we move to embrace the fullness of life as God intended. My fellow students who have read and re-read this book and kept God's Word active in their lives have powerful testimonies of personal healing and growth.

It is my hope that as you benefit from the principles in this book, that you will spread the word to small groups, churches and communities across America and beyond.

I have conducted many weekly group studies in my home . Groups were as small as eight and sometimes as large as fourteen. Each meeting ran as long as it needed to so that we could meet the specific needs of each participant.

A typical meeting began with 15 minutes of sharing, followed by 45 minutes of study and occasional excerpts from various DVD series. "It's a New Day" by Henry and Donna Wright was a favorite.[1] Sometimes we dedicated entire evenings to reading, studying, and praying aloud.

In proving these principles, we regularly witnessed personal growth and physical transformations, resulting in new testimonies each session. As we took God's promises seriously, we gained inspiration, faith, and healing.

Our central theme: growing in relationship with God, conforming to His teachings, and realizing the amazing gift and power of verbal prayer, Scripture, commands, and proclamation over our entire being and health challenges.

As these study groups evolved over time, I added portions of the DVD series "The Seven Pillars of Health" when addressing the section on Physical Health, and principles of Carolyn Leaf's DVD "Your Body, His Temple" when moving through the Mental Health section. I also like Keith Moore's DVD's. (See Endnotes for ordering information.) You are certainly not limited to these tools. There is plenty of complimentary information available from sources on the Internet and in bookstores.

In beginning this study, your greatest potential is with God's blessing. Here are a few questions for consideration:

1. Have you accepted God's loving invitation for adoption as His child? This is the Gospel of Salvation or "Good News" of the Bible (Appendix I). This is an amazing honor He has offered us and He has created a great owner's manual as our guide.

2. Please ask yourself: Do I truly want to get well and move toward full alignment in spiritual health (which includes my physical, mental, emotional, and spiritual energies)? Sometimes we are attached to our current situation and the attention we receive while in it. Proclaiming your intention aloud to become well sends a message to your ears, brain, and into every portion of your being that it is time for change!

"I am ready today to release ALL of my pain and trauma, and all attached stories related to all of my physical, mental, emotional, and spiritual concerns. I am ready to truly

learn and embark upon a journey of discovery and wellness, clearing out all obstacles in my path!"

3. Are you willing to take the time needed for true and lasting change? I have been incorporating these principles in my life for years and am still undergoing exciting changes. Be patient. Persevere until you have mastery over this material. It took awhile to arrive at where you are and just the same, it takes time to change.

This journey will require faith (the ability to believe what is not yet seen) and action, as is often the case with any new and worthwhile endeavor.

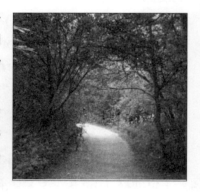

We will examine unprofitable habits, thoughts, emotions, and patterns that bind us to disease and hoard the spaces that precious pearls of health are meant to occupy.

Ready to begin? On this journey, you will discover God's willingness to be your trustworthy guide.

Your word is a lamp to my feet and a light to my path (Ps 119:105).

Prepare Yourself for Effective, Victorious Prayer

The Bible likens accepting God's invitation of salvation to accepting an invitation to a sumptuous marriage feast. Many of God's promises are conditional upon accepting this invitation. You do not have to wait until everything is perfect in your life. Life is never perfect. Challenges and obstacles always lay along life's path. Step forward in faith and each additional step will only add more strength, skill, and confidence.

When desiring God's promises and blessings, we must be humble and obedient when coming before Him to speak and pray in the power of Jesus' name. Preparing ourselves before we engage in serious prayer is always wise.

Start by confessing any known sin in your spiritual journey that is robbing you of intimacy with God. Declare your intention to align your entire being to God's will. State your resistance to Satan and his mind games.

Second, forgive anyone toward whom you have resentment or bitterness. Do this in person or out loud in a private place.

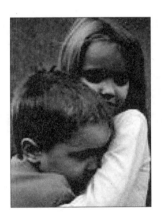

Lessons from children —

the peaceful fruits of forgiveness.

Make an ongoing commitment to repent (turn aside from) any sin of which you are aware so that it does not enslave you. Verbally invite and affirm God as your counselor, healer, and guide.

Therefore submit to God. Resist the devil and he will flee from you. Draw near to God and He will draw near to you. Cleanse your hands, you sinners; and purify your hearts, you double-minded (James 4:7-8).

And whenever you stand praying, if you have anything against anyone, forgive him that your Father in heaven may also forgive your trespasses. But if you do not forgive, neither will your Father in heaven forgive your trespasses (Mark 11:25-26).

Now, invite God to make your life a masterpiece in progress! Thank Him in advance for providing and beginning the healing of your physical, emotional, mental, and spiritual wounds. Share with Him the intentions of your heart. Daily visualize and feel the weaving together of your tapestry of complete healing. Make a visual chart of your goals. Expect your relationship with God to blossom as you align with the pearls of truth that follow.

For we are His workmanship, created in Christ Jesus for good works, which God prepared beforehand that we should walk in them (Eph 2:10).

Being confident of this very thing, that He who has begun a good work in you will complete it until the day of Jesus Christ (Phil 1:6).

Beloved, I pray that you may prosper in all things and be in health, just as your soul prospers. I have no greater joy than to hear that my children walk in truth (3 John 1:2,4).

This should make clear that God's will is for you to be in health. But we have responsibilities in this also.

God requires integrity, that is, aligning His truth with our thinking, speaking, and actions as well as our thoughts, emotions, diet and lifestyle.

With these in balance, we experience peace and our highest health potential.

The following chart is a great visual that can help us begin to implement these principles.

Take some time to meditate and pray on how you believe God wants you to grow in these areas.

PERSONAL GOALS FOR THIS STUDY: _____

_____
_____
_____
_____
_____
_____
_____
_____
_____
_____
_____
_____
_____
_____
_____
_____
_____
_____
_____
_____

Please personalize the following chart. Copy it and place it where you can see it daily.

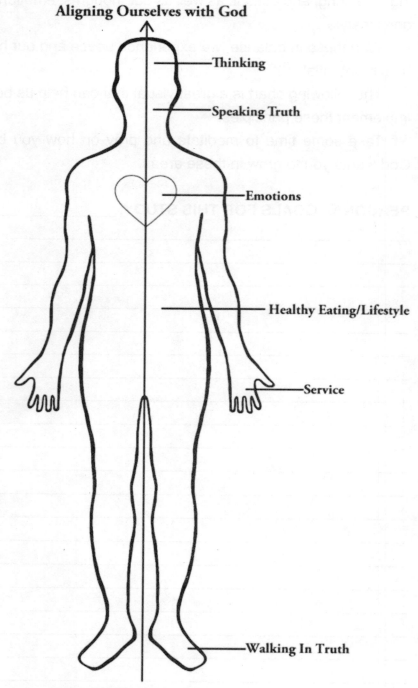

Aligning Ourselves with God

Thinking

Speaking Truth

Emotions

Healthy Eating/Lifestyle

Service

Walking In Truth

Is the Recipe for Joy

Illustrated by Catherine Drauch

Part 1
Pearls of Physical Health

P HYSICAL HEATH: a state in which we enjoy a human body that functions as optimally as possible. It rebuilds, heals, and energizes itself properly. It cleanses and drains metabolic and environmental toxins efficiently so that they exit through the eliminative channels of the colon, kidneys, skin, and lungs. When the body is healthy, it functions as God intended.

In God's Word, Jesus warns that there is a battle between good and evil (the "thief") over what God made.

The thief does not come except to steal, and to kill, and to destroy. I have come that they may have life, and that they may have it more abundantly (John 10:10).

Know your enemy. Satan and his dark forces have infiltrated this world and prowl like lions looking for prey, to destroy or steal anything we have left unprotected.

His self-appointed mission is to shorten our lives with destructive

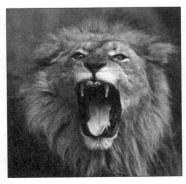

habits, and barrage us with tempting, health-destroying thoughts, hoping we will adopt them as our own. He aims to steal our health and our joy and make us miserable and ineffective.

The Scriptures state that our battle is not with each other but with the dark forces within the spiritual realms that continually attempt to obtain a foothold in our lives. The targets: our bodies, minds, emotions, and spirits. Satan desires to kill, steal, and destroy all that is precious to God. His name means the accuser.

He hurls accusation against us, God, and all that God teaches when we yield to the destructive enticements that run us off the road to true life and health. Don't settle for living in the ditch.

Evaluate all choices, thoughts, and emotions that enter your consciousness. Our goal is to reject accusing and destructive thoughts toward ourselves, others, God, and anything else not rooted in God's truth.

Take up your pearls that Jesus offers. Use them as your armor, weapons, and a means of discernment. With these in place, you become a being of power and strength, rendering Satan powerless.

Do not give ground to anything that can steal your health at any level. It is a precious gift to be guarded carefully.

HEALING PEARL:
WE NEED KNOWLEDGE

Too many of God's people today are plagued with all sorts of diseases, despite their access to Biblical tools complete for every good work. Ignorant of basic health principles, millions suffer unnecessarily and die prematurely.

On what day of the week did God create disease? He called

His creation "good." Disease then is a by-product of 'missing the mark.' God wants us back on track.

My people are destroyed for lack of knowledge
(Hosea 4:6).

We consume food that is processed, sprayed, irradiated, canned, refined, preserved, and genetically altered. We build and furnish our homes with materials that emit toxic, poisonous gases. Many of our creams, lotions, and shampoos have little natural components, and are loaded with chemicals.

We cleanse our clothes and home with toxic chemical concoctions that act as a type of chemical estrogen, confusing our bodies and throwing them off-balance. We contaminate our water with toxic chemicals, pesticides, and heavy metals.

We pollute our air with metals, soot, chemicals, and electromagnetic frequencies from cell phones and their towers.

When ill, our traditional treatments often involve cutting, irradiating, and ingesting even more chemicals.

If a space traveler from another planet landed here and mingled with us for awhile, he might get the impression that we are obsessed with the use of poisons! This is mankind's doing. In the beginning, it was not this way.

HEALING PEARL:
DIETARY PRINCIPLES OF THE BIBLE

When God first made mankind, He also made the perfect diet—a diet rich in raw, organic food and pure water.

And God said, "See, I have given you every herb that yields seed which is on the face of all the earth, and every tree whose fruit yields seed; to you it shall be for food (Gen 1:29).

The term "herb" pertains to vegetation —both nutritional and medicinal. These are fruits, vegetables, grains, nuts, and seeds. God, later, introduces the option of eating animal protein.

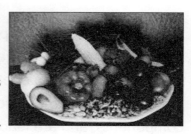

Just as the longevity and proper running of your car depends on proper care, fuel, and maintenance, so does your body. Its health is directly related to certain physical laws and principles. God, in His goodness and as our Designer, patiently teaches these. His way is not the world's way. We are to be an example of true abundant living. We must become open-minded to change and willing to receive instruction.

And do not be conformed to this world, but be transformed by the renewing of your mind, that you may prove what is that good and acceptable and perfect will of God (Rom 12:2).

All Scripture is given by inspiration of God, and is profitable for doctrine, for reproof, for correction, for instruction in righteousness [...] (2 Tim 3:16).

Our health habits are important. Everything we do or neglect to do has positive or negative consequences.

Do not be deceived, God is not mocked; for whatever a

man sows, this he will also reap (Gal 6:7).

In the Old Testament, God chose a people (the Israelites) who were to obey His teaching and represent His goodness and truth. The Scriptures note that the Israelites, even while slaves in Egypt were physically hardy. What was their health secret?

We remember the fish which we ate freely in Egypt, the cucumbers, the melons, the leeks, the onions, and the garlic... (Num 11:5).

- **Fish:** In Dr. Harold Manner's book, "The Death of Cancer," fish is the only flesh product allowed for one who is ill with certain degenerative diseases.[4] It is easy to digest and rich in heart and brain-nourishing omega-3 oils.

- **Cucumber:** nourishing to the complexion, hair, digestion, and kidneys. It may ease inflammation and heat in the body through its cooling action.

- **Melons:** a natural diuretic and kidney food that is rich in vitamins A and C. Its energy may also cool inflamed tissues.

- **Leeks, onions, and garlic:** rich in organic sulfur, which assists the cells in detoxification. These foods may nourish the joints and circulation, build stamina, and assist the body in the reduction of opportunistic organisms, such as yeasts and parasites.

And the midwives said to Pharaoh, "Because the Hebrew women are not as the Egyptian women; for they are vigorous, and they give birth before the midwife can get to them" (Ex 1:19, New American Standard Bible®).

The Israelites grew up eating healthy, unprocessed, organic food. More importantly, their faith and trust resided in the promises of God. God called them *His* people. As He gathered the Israelites to Himself and brought them out of Egypt, He gave them a promise:

[...] If you diligently heed the voice of the LORD your God and do what is right in His sight, give ear to His commandments and keep all His statutes, I will put none of the diseases on you which I have brought on the Egyptians for I am the LORD who heals you (Ex 15:26).

Did you notice that this is a conditional promise? Note what role God was willing to fulfill and, I believe, is still willing to fulfill for those who follow Him today.

Do you want God on your healing team? Commit to doing His will. Raise your hands to the Lord. Ask Him to take the seat of honor. He awaits your invitation.

I will therefore that men pray everywhere, lifting up holy hands [...] (I Tim 2:8).

Moses was one hundred and twenty years old when he died. His eyes were not dim nor his natural vigor diminished (Deut 34:7).

Moses, a great man of God and called the most humble of men in the Old Testament, was a leader of the Israelites. He lived to be one hundred and twenty years old.

His successor, Joshua, was vigorous, full of faith, and confident in the face of overwhelming opposition at the age of eighty-five:

> And now, behold, the LORD has kept me alive, as He said, these forty-five years, ever since the LORD spoke this word to Moses while Israel wandered in the wilderness; and now, here I am this day, eighty-five years old. As yet I am as strong this day as on the day that Moses sent me; just as my strength was then, so now is my strength for war, both for going out and for coming in. Now therefore, give me this mountain of which the LORD spoke in that day; for you heard in that day how the Anakim were there, and that the cities were great and fortified. It may be that the LORD will be with me, and I shall be able to drive them out as the LORD said (Josh 14:10-12).

Moses and Joshua were both enviable in their old age for their vigor and health. How do you intend to feel when you are eighty-five?

I want to make it clear that I do not believe that God condemns us for what we eat today--that is, I do not believe it is a test of our salvation. However, I will ask you to consider that God, as a Master of Creation, is also a Master Nutritionist and knows what type of diet is best for our physical health.

Dr. Rex Russell, M.D. was a physician afflicted with diabetes for twenty-five years. His symptoms included chronic abscesses, arthritis, leg swelling, artery deterioration, and eyesight and kidney afflictions. After rounds of medications as well as natural supplements, he carefully studied and decided to try God's master diet plan given to the Israelites.

His results: a gradual falling away of the majority of his symptoms, including complete eradication of his arthritis. If you wish to read the inspirational story of Rex Russel, it is present in his book, *What the Bible Says About Healthy Living.*[2]

The following outline is only a portion of God's plan for the physical health of the Israelites. God wanted them to be a holy people, set apart from the other nations, not just spiritually, but also in the way that they ate. Consider experimenting with these principles, especially if you have health challenges.

A valuable rule of health is to eat the Creator's food in the most pure state that you can. Avoid messing with it too much. This means avoiding most processed, boxed, and canned foods. Eat what you can raw or lightly steamed, sautéed, or broiled, and avoid deep-frying. Use oils like olive, virgin coconut, grape seed, and sesame -- especially when you need to heat them for cooking. Utilize herbs for seasoning, as well as raw apple vinegar, fresh lemon juice and zest, and unrefined salt. Keeping food simple, organic, and pure is a key to vibrant heath.

Living with Knowledge: Principles of Health in Leviticus 11

- **Eat, as much as possible, non-genetically modified, fresh organic vegetables, fruits, nuts, grains, and seeds**. By definition, this will also include herbs. They are shown scientifically to be a great match for our type of teeth and digestive tract. Gorillas eat a similar diet and have digestive systems most comparable to ours.

- **Eat only "clean" meat.** Ideally these should be organically raised. Biblically "clean" animals have both a divided hoof and chew cud, e.g. cattle, lamb, sheep, goat, and venison.

- **Do not eat "unclean" meat.** This will include cat, dog, camel, rabbit, bear, horse, squirrel, opossum, weasel, rat, guinea pig, pig, lizard, chameleon, gecko, skunk and anything else that does not qualify.

- **Eat "clean" fowl.** Examples are chicken, turkey, geese, duck, quail, and pigeon.

- **Do not eat "unclean" fowl.** Examples are vulture, raven, hawk, owl, eagle, osprey, crow, heron, bat, ostrich, seagull, stork, and pelican.

- **Eat "clean" fish. They must have fins and scales.** A few examples are salmon, sea bass, tuna, sole, haddock, halibut, bluefish, perch, smelt, trout, herring, flounder, cod, and flying fish. Goldfish also qualify, if you are tempted.

- **Do not eat "unclean" fish.** Some examples are stingray, scallops, oysters, catfish, crab, eel, octopus, scallops, lobster, crawfish, squid, puffer fish, shark, shrimp, and clams. Today, shelled bottom feeders are more likely to accumulate and concentrate within their bodies chemicals and metals that sink to the bottom of oceans, rivers, and streams.

- For those of you who thrive on adventure, you may also eat **"clean" insects** that are winged, hop, and have four legs, such as locusts, grasshoppers, and crickets.

- **You must not eat "unclean" bugs and insects,** which basically include everything else.

  This is the law of the animals and the birds, and every living creature that moves in the waters, and of every creature that creeps on the earth, To distinguish between the unclean and the clean, and between the animal that may be eaten and the animal that may not be eaten (Lev 11:46,47).

Most churches teach today that all foods are now permitted due to current mainstream interpretations of the New Testament teachings. However, the Seventh Day Adventists, who still choose to eat according to Old Testament dietary principles, are scientifically noted for their superior longevity.

Again, it may not be a sin to eat all food types freely, but it may not be in our best interests if we desire optimal health.

Let us examine a few more foods from God's word that science agrees are highly nutritious:

For the LORD your God is bringing you into a good land, a land of brooks of water, of fountains and springs, that flow out of valleys and hills; a land of wheat and barley, of vines and fig trees and pomegranates, a land of olive oil and honey (Deut 8:7-8).

- **Wheat:** the original wheat, today known as spelt or kamut, was not a hybrid like most of today's wheat, which seems to be causing a rash of gluten intolerance in many people. Consider eating soaked and sprouted whole grains, which are easier to digest and may be less allergenic.

- **Barley:** easily digested and drought and insect resistant. It contains excellent nutrients for the body to promote healthy cholesterol levels. Consider as a highly nutritious addition to soups.

- **Grapes:** an excellent blood and immune builder. Its seeds contain a powerful antioxidant more than twenty times the power of Vitamin C or E. Johanna Brandt details her fascinating recovery from cancer using whole concord grapes in her book, "The Grape Cure."[3]

- **Figs:** a nutritious, soothing food for the intestinal tract.

- **Pomegranates:** rich in ellagic acid. This powerful cell protector is studied for its properties that may inhibit chemically induced cancers as well as trigger cell death in cancer cells in the laboratory.

- **Olive oil:** one of the healthiest oils. Olive oil and lemon juice have long been used by herbalists to promote healthy liver and gallbladder function and to assist the normal fluidity of the blood. Olive oil is friendly to the digestion and circulation. Healthy oils promote a healthy healing response.

- **Raw Honey:** the only sweetener mentioned in the Bible. Honey has antibiotic properties and has been used to topically prevent infections in wounds. It contains chromium, a mineral required to help process sugars. Royal jelly,

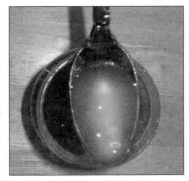

found in honeycomb, may be powerful for the support of healthy hormones, endurance, healing, and fertility. Honey, a concentrated sweetener, is to be eaten sparingly-- a wise principle to apply to all sweets.

Have you found honey? Eat only as much as you need, lest you be filled with it and vomit (Prov 25:16).

Did you know that in some desserts, like a banana split, we can consume twenty-five teaspoons of sugar? However, we cannot easily eat the same amount in honey. When we consume sweets in their natural form, our body knows when to stop. There is a natural gag reflex. With refined sugars, that natural reflex is often absent or delayed, as these sugars are foreign to the body's design. Too frequently this results in the consumption of massive amounts of sugar that are harmful to our bodies.

Our blood stream holds approximately one teaspoon of sugar when our blood sugar is in normal range. If we consume more than one to two teaspoons at a sitting, we risk our fat cells plumping up with the excess sugar. Our cell walls may become inflamed, setting the stage for disease processes to begin.

The Bible is rich in exciting, profitable pearls that teach us about healthy foods and how we may enjoy vibrant health. God wants us to be healthy and wise in our food choices.

God's Bread Recipe

Did you know that there is a bread recipe in the Bible?

Also take for yourself wheat, barley, beans, lentils, millet, and spelt; put them into one vessel, and make bread of them for yourself. During the number of days that you lie on your side, three hundred and ninety days, you shall eat it (Ezek 4:9).

This is a bread recipe that can truly support life and health! Some local health-food stores sell breads and cereals that contain some or all of these health ingredients. Two examples are Ezekiel bread and Ezekiel cereal.

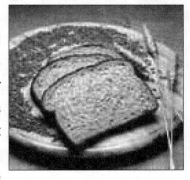

Unleavened bread is easier for some to digest and may result in less bloating and indigestion, as it does not contain yeast or high gluten levels. Consider gluten-free bread if you have digestive, immune, or joint challenges.

(Photo courtesy of the Wheat Foods Council)

Now the woman had a fatted calf in the house, and she hastened to kill it. And she took flour and kneaded it, and baked unleavened bread from it (1 Sam 28:24).

In the Bible, people did not make or eat genetically-altered grain or refined bread with preservatives. Today we refine flour by taking out about twenty-six nutrients and putting approximately eight back in. From this flour, we make "enriched" bread. How enriched would you be if your dentist pulled twenty-six teeth and reimplanted eight?

Throughout the Scriptures, wholesome, organic, unrefined bread is a symbol of high-quality sustenance—physically and spiritually. Buy with discernment your bread, crackers, cereals, and chips.

The Eating of Blood and Fat

In the time of Noah, God had specific dietary instructions. This was before any of the dietary laws given to the Israelites.

> But you shall not eat flesh with its life, that is, its blood (Gen 9:4).

God has sound reasons for all his commands, though He may not share them with us. He wants us to trust him and be obedient through faith. We already know that blood can carry a multitude of infections as well as microscopic parasites. Science only recently has been able to isolate the AIDS virus in some samples of blood. More mysteries about blood and what it carries might be solved in the future.

> And the LORD spoke to Moses, saying, "Speak to the children of Israel, saying, 'You shall not eat any fat, of ox or sheep or goat (Lev 7:23,24).

We now know that the saturated fat of animals is a hard fat and difficult for our bodies to process. Fat is also a storage place for chemical solvents, antibiotics, insecticides, and feed hormones. These hard, cover fats can be some of the most toxic of tissues in the animal. Saturated fats today are associated with various cancers, heart and blood vessel disease, obesity, and more.

HEALING PEARL:
THE PRINCIPLE OF FOOD QUALITY

Today, there is a broad range of food quality within our supermarkets. Avoid items of poor nutrient quality and those contaminated by toxic environments, such as some fish. God desires us to eat high-quality, nutritious food as opposed to empty, calorie-laden junk food. The sound spiritual principle below is easily applied to our physical health.

Why do you spend money for what is not bread, and your wages for what does not satisfy? Listen carefully to Me, and eat what is good, and let your soul delight itself in abundance (Isa 55:2).

The following principle may suggest that God approves of the spending of extra time or travel to select quality foods for our families. Be selective in what you purchase.

Who can find a virtuous wife? For her worth is far above rubies. She is like the merchant ships, she brings her food from afar (Prov 31:10,14).

HEALING PEARL:
THE PRINCIPLE OF WATER QUALITY

A fountain of gardens, a well of living waters, and streams from Lebanon (Song 4:15).

For the LORD your God is bringing you into a good land, a land of brooks of water, of fountains and springs that flow out of valleys and hills (Deut 8:7).

The Bible speaks favorably of quality water. In the first verse, the context refers to the enjoyment and value of fresh, pure water and how it is used to compliment the attributes of a beautiful woman. In the latter, water is one of the blessings involved in God's plan for His people.

Currently, water is polluted with man-made additives and a variety of toxic chemicals coming from industries. These toxins may store in vulnerable organs and tissues in our bodies, causing inflammation and disease. Because of this, as well as the seepage of pesticides into the ground water beneath wells, a high-quality water purifier is a worthy investment as it can remove harmful particles, leaving water once again in a pure, clean state.[5]

Almost everything we eat contains an element of water. There is some amazing and extremely compelling evidence that our prayers, thoughts, intentions, and words contain and emit energies that imprint easily upon water. What if we could literally program the water or food we eat before we consume it?

Could we program our water by holding and praying that it become a therapeutic agent for specific health challenges? Could giving thanks over our food and water change it energetically so that it becomes more health promoting? These are interesting and thought-provoking questions to consider.

If this interests you, read about related experiments in the fascinating book, "The True Power of Water," by Masaru Emoto.[6]

See how Judi and Jon have used the power of water to their advantage when holding some water-based solutions that they wished to improve:

JUDI'S PRAYER

Heavenly Father, through your Son, Jesus Christ, and the power of the Holy Spirit, we believe that you already sent your special healing power through this fluid.

We believe you infused this fluid with compatibility, love, thankfulness, relaxation, calmness, good grace, peace of mind, relief, compassion, ... tolerance, pleasure, joy and gratitude.

We praise and thank you for already making this fluid heal my body in the right way. I pray any and all contaminants be wholly, completely neutralized, and rendered harmless to my body. We believe this healing prayer already accomplished what it was supposed to. Amen.

This testimony is from a cancer survivor who received monthly, filtered blood infusions by IV. Frequently, she related that she reacted violently to each. In an effort to lessen this response, her doctor prescribed anti-allergy medication. This went on for several months. Even so, she still stated that she felt ill and took days to recover. Then she read the book, The True Power of Water, by Masaru Emoto, which shares evidence that we can influence fluid-based items with the God-given frequencies and energies within words. We discussed the possibility of her and her husband holding and praying verbally over the IV just before the infusion while holding the bottle. Judi stated that her doctor noticed such a difference that he began to double-check that she and her husband had prayed before the treatment began.

JON'S PRAYER

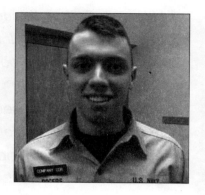

Heavenly Father, I pray and command, in Jesus' name, that all elements of this anthrax vaccine be blessed to the good of my body and that any toxic elements or contaminants within it be neutralized and rendered as nontoxic as water within my system.

I claim this in faith and belief in the amazing power of God. With God, nothing is impossible! I claim the Lord as my primary healer and physician.

Thank you, Lord. I pray this in Jesus' name. Amen.

Jon asked permission to pray over his military vaccine and received it. He stepped aside from the line of men, held the vaccine, and verbally prayed over it, commanding its use to be for his health only. The anthrax vaccine is known to cause intense burning when injected. Jon had no burning at all. The medic was amazed.

Speaking over anything containing liquid with positive intentional words creates energetic change. Consider speaking not only over foods and liquids that you will be exposed to but also over your own body which is 80% water. You can greatly influence your health with this amazing gift from God.

HEALING PEARL
THE PRINCIPLE OF SELF-CONTROL

Self-control is a powerful principle of health. I believe that when we violate this, we set ourselves up for many diseases, including diabetes, heart disease, cancer, obesity and a host of digestive ailments.

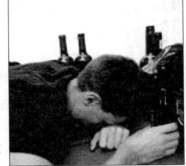

Everyone could benefit from not eating to excess or over-indulging in items that may be addictive, such as white sugar, coffee, soda, cigarettes, and alcohol.

All things are lawful for me, but all things are not helpful. All things are lawful for me, but I will not be brought under the power of any (1 Cor 6:12).

Whoever has no rule over his own spirit is like a city broken down, without walls (Prov 25:28).

And they shall say to the elders of his city, "This son of ours is stubborn and rebellious; he will not obey our voice; he is a glutton and a drunkard" (Deut 21:20).

Our appetites and cravings are not to dictate our diets nor the amounts we consume. Food and drink are not to become our masters. When we overindulge in rich foods, addictive foods, or junk foods, we run risks. Self-control is never as limiting to personal freedom as disease is.

We now know scientifically how important healthy foods are to our bodies. Researchers around the world are studying longevity-promoting foods and lifestyles, with a heavy focus on the Mediterranean diet, the healthy diets of the elderly Okinawans and Costa Ricans, and others. For more about these locations known for their longevity, research The Blue Zones.[7]

HEALING PEARL:
EATING IN A POSITIVE ATMOSPHERE

A pleasant atmosphere is always suggested when eating alone or with others. You may have to turn off the news.

Better is a dinner of herbs where love is, than a fatted calf with hatred (Prov 15:17).

Better is a dry morsel with quietness, than a house full of feasting with strife (Prov 17:1).

Better to dwell in a corner of a housetop, than in a house shared with a contentious woman (Prov 21:9).
(Or man, for that matter.)

Our digestive processes become stressed when we become stressed. Our digestive juices will not secrete properly when we are under the influence of upsetting emotions and thoughts, leading to over-acidity, fermentation, and putrefaction of the food within our intestines. Gas, bloating, indigestion, and even ulcers may result. The antacid and indigestion medication industry is a multi-billion dollar business in the United States today.

HEALING PEARL:
THOUGHTS AND EMOTIONS AFFECT OUR BODIES, ESPECIALLY OUR BONES

Do not be wise in your own eyes; fear the LORD and depart from evil. It will be health to your flesh, and strength to your bones (Prov 3:7-8).

A sound heart is life to the body, but envy is rottenness to the bones (Prov 14:30).

The light of the eyes rejoices the heart, and a good report makes the bones healthy (Prov 15:30).

Pleasant words are like honeycomb, sweetness to the soul and health to the bones (Prov 16:24).

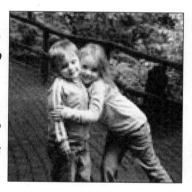

A merry heart does good, like medicine, but a broken spirit dries the bones (Prov 17:22).

A large part of our immunity resides within our bones, particularly in the bone marrow where stem cells are made.

HEALING PEARL:
FOODS, HERBS, AND ESSENTIAL OILS ARE TOOLS FOR HEALING

Now Isaiah had said, "Let them take a lump of figs, and apply it as a poultice on the boil, and he shall recover (Isa 38:21).

Purge me with hyssop, and I shall be clean; wash me, and I shall be whiter than snow (Ps 51:7).

Then they gave Him wine mingled with myrrh to drink, but He did not take it (Mark 15:23).

In Mark 15, Jesus was offered myrrh, a painkiller, while on the cross. Myrrh can be both an essential oil and an herbal extract.

The people of the Bible had a good understanding of God's pharmacy stocked with herbs and essential oils. They used these natural remedies for daily health and healing. In Psalms 51, King David references hyssop when speaking of his spiritual need for God and forgiveness. Hyssop is known in herbal medicine as an excellent internal body purifier.

Similar symbolism is used when describing God's provision:

Along the bank of the river, on this side and that, will grow all kinds of trees used for food; their leaves will not wither, and their fruit will not fail. They will bear fruit every month, because their water flows from the sanctuary. Their fruit will be for food, and their leaves for medicine (Ezek 47:12).

Herbs are medicinal and/or nutritional plants. They have been used extensively since the beginning of time and have a great safety record compared to medications. For thousands of years in India and China, herbs have been recorded as medicinal tools in primary health care. They are rich in nutrients that build and strengthen tissues and organs as well as loosen and drain toxins. For example, the beautiful passion flower has been historically used internally to calm an over-active mind and strengthen the eyes. Herbs are legally classified as foods in the United States.

He causeth the grass to grow for the cattle, and (the) herb for the service of man [...] (Ps 104:14, KJV).

God approves of our use of herbs. Western medicine has also discovered their value and attempts to retain this value when refining them. However, isolated chemical compounds used as drugs for patent lose the natural buffers of the whole plant, leaving the potential for harmful side effects.

Pharmaceutical drugs have saved many lives and there is a time and place for them. However, many people have found effective and safer alternatives by utilizing the unrefined herbs that God created.

Essential oils, an aromatic concentrated component from plants and flowers, are highly therapeutic, absorb easily through the skin, and can enter the entire blood stream in seconds. They are used as powerful tools to trigger physical, mental, and emotional healing.

Essential oils are different from and far more potent therapeutically than our grocery store vegetable oils and are favorably cited in the Scriptures.

> *To console those who mourn in Zion, to give them beauty for ashes, the oil of joy for mourning (Isa 61:3).*

> *All your garments are scented with myrrh and aloes and cassia, out of the ivory palaces, by which they have made you glad (Ps 45:8).*

I love these verses, because they associate essential oils with healthy emotional states. Many health practitioners today use essential oils such as lavender, rose, frankincense, neroli, jasmine, and rosemary, to ease the effects of depression, anxiety, grief, and more.

> *Your plants are an orchard of pomegranates with pleasant fruits, fragrant henna with spikenard, spikenard and saffron, calamus and cinnamon, with all trees of frankincense, myrrh and aloes, with all the chief spices [...]*
> *(Song 4:13-14).*

> *And when they had come into the house, they saw the young Child with Mary His mother, and fell down and worshiped Him. And when they had opened their treasures, they presented gifts to Him: gold, frankincense, and myrrh (Matt 2:11).*

I have observed many people who have used both herbs and essential oils for healing after exhausting their medical options. God references highly valued herbs and essential oils to symbolize His goodness. There are two hundred and twenty-three references to the use of oils in the New King James Version of the Bible. Their usage is recorded throughout the Old Testament, up through the time of Christ. They are one of the oldest forms of medicine and cosmetics known to man. Historically, some were considered more valuable than gold. Health practitioners are still investigating their unique properties today.

As for the herbal and essential oil industry, it is growing by leaps and bounds as people discover their wonderful benefits. Their products are extremely affordable and safe when properly used.

Essential oils are fifty to seventy times the concentration of most herbs. They are generally used externally on the skin in small amounts, in baths, and as aromatherapy. It is important to use them with caution and knowledge. Essential oil expert, Dr. D. Gary Young, states, "People using essential oils have a sixty percent greater resistance to illness. Not only that, but when using essential oils, they may recover seventy percent faster from a given illness."[8]

Historical Uses of Essential Oils Mentioned in the Bible

Myrrh is popularly used to support immunity and repel infectious organisms. It is valued for fungal skin conditions and rashes. It may be used to assist the respiratory system and the mucus membranes when infected or sore, especially the gums. It also is used for digestive and prostate support.

Hyssop is taught to have anti-inflammatory, anti-scarring, and antiviral properties. It is reported to assist the discharge of toxins and mucus from the respiratory system.

Frankincense is used therapeutically in European hospitals to release mucus and ease scarring. It has been used as an anti-tumor agent, immune-stimulator, and mood elevator -- stimulating and elevating the mind, thereby lifting the mood.

Cinnamon bark oil has at least a two thousand-year history of use in Sri Lanka. It is historically used to fight infections and viruses. Because cinnamon bark is a spicy "hot" oil, it is best diluted with vegetable oils before application to the skin.

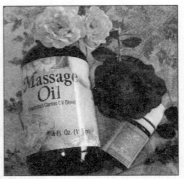

All essential oils may be diluted in a massage oil blend for easy application to large areas of the body.

I have personally found that applying essential oils, mostly undiluted, to the bottom of my feet and also to my spine has had amazing benefits in assisting my body to cool itself, align my spine, release trauma, and more.

I have also had multiple client feedback regarding how their bodies repaired their knees and shoulders while using the daily application of both Nature's Sunshine Tei-fu oil lotion (about one half teaspoon) and clove oil (about five to ten drops) for one to two months.

Essential oils have the power to assist the body in breaking up tough patterns of imbalance, thereby making them an invaluable part of a healthy lifestyle.

HEALING PEARL:
THE PRINCIPLE OF PERSEVERANCE

Have you ever been tempted to give up and accept mediocre health because you have not received your desired results? Perhaps it is time to implement a few new available tools.

Prescription medicine is only one piece of the pie. There is much more to investigate.

Today, Western medicine, with pharmaceuticals as its primary tool, has become a dominating force due to its giant political lobby in the United States. Synthetic drugs, in general, have no nutritional content. Their side effects may be similar to the sickness or disorders that they are designed to treat. Many cause nutrient deficiencies and negatively interact with other drugs.

Deaths from pharmaceuticals and their side effects are now at an estimated seven hundred and eighty-four thousand per year.[9] With this in mind, serious prayer and investigation should be undertaken in regard to any long-term use. Many have searched out and found safer alternatives in the field of natural medicine.

Most medications focus on the symptoms, not the cause. For those who have been told there is no cure, remember this is often proclaimed within a specific framework of pharmaceutical education. Be responsible for your health—educate yourself and ask questions. Investigate why herbs, essential oils, and other natural remedies are exploding in popularity.

Note: some medications do not mix well with herbs or essential oils. Ask your pharmacist.

God supports the principle of perseverance, and we can apply it to our health. Disease is not a blessing, and we should not be content to simply endure it before seeking out possible physical, emotional, mental, and spiritual causes. We are told to be a people of faith, boldness, and

Dr. Christopher, courtesy of the School of Natural Health

persistence. If one door closes, look for another one to open.

Dr. John Christopher, a great pioneering Master Herbalist of his day, passionately taught that our loving God created natural remedies for every disease known to man.[11]

I remember when he described the case of a young boy who suffered painful, third degree burns on both of his hands. He had two medical choices: skin grafts that would severely impair movement of the hand or amputation. His parents decided to first seek an alternative herbal option. Dr. Christopher made a paste of equal parts ground fresh comfrey, wheat germ oil, and raw honey and gave instructions to apply it fresh daily and not to wash it off. He intended the mixture to feed the tissue externally, and he had his desired result. The boy's hand, including the skin, healed completely with full function. Even the fingernails grew back.

Are you searching for new doors to open? God may bring an answer that you may not expect. Be open to alternative paths. Investigate. Do not give up! Persist and persevere.

And He said to them, "Which of you shall have a friend, and go to him at mid-night and say to him, 'Friend, lend me three loaves; for a friend of mine has come to me on his journey, and I have nothing to set before him'; and he will answer from within and say, 'Do not trouble me; the door is now shut, and my children are with me in bed; I cannot rise and give to you'? I say to you, though he will not rise and give to him because he is his friend, yet because of his persistence he will rise and give him as many as he needs. So I say

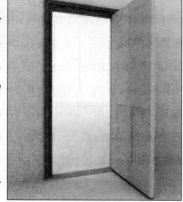

to you, ask, and it will be given to you; seek, and you will find; knock, and it will be opened to you. For everyone who asks receives, and he who seeks finds, and to him who knocks it will be opened" (Luke 11:5-10).

This woman in the Bible had all doors to healing closed to her:

Now a certain woman had a flow of blood for twelve years, and had suffered many things from many physicians. She had spent all that she had and was no better, but rather grew worse (Mark 5:25-26).

Suffering, mounting medical bills, bankruptcy, etc. Sounds like a typical day in America. This persistent woman's story continues:

When she heard about Jesus, she came behind Him in the crowd and touched His garment; for she said, "If only I may touch His clothes, I shall be made well." Immediately the fountain of her blood was dried up, and she felt in her body that she was healed of the affliction [...] And He said to her, "Daughter, your faith has made you well. Go in peace, and be healed of your affliction" (Mark 5:27-29,34).

This woman's faith and willingness to explore new possibilities resulted in a new lease on life.

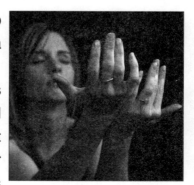

Our opportunities and answers often come through unexpected sources. Examine all doors that present themselves when you are praying for answers. Have faith in a God who is a master at making a door out of a wall. Thousands have found answers this way.

Below I have summarized two major avenues of scriptural healing that involve trusting in God's provisions. If you are ready to try something new, the next precious pearls are waiting.

HEALING PEARL:
A SUPERNATURAL APPROACH TO HEALING

Meditate on clearing your conscience. Repent of any sins committed knowingly and unknowingly. Verbally release all unforgiveness. We can block God's blessing by participating in sin. Pray, possibly with fasting (please make sure beforehand that you can medically do this), for God's assistance in your healing. It is certainly permissible to ask God for a creative miracle. Enlist others to pray over you and with you.

For where two or three are gathered together in My name, I am there in the midst of them (Matt 18:20).

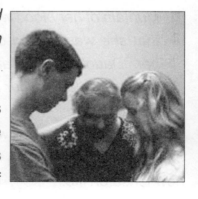

You may also wish to go to the elders of the church for prayer. Notice the importance of clearing one's conscience when seeking this form of healing:

Is anyone among you sick? Let him call for the elders of the church, and let them pray over him, anointing him with oil in the name of the Lord. And the prayer of faith will save the sick, and the Lord will raise him up. And if he has committed sins, he will be forgiven. Confess your trespasses to one another, and pray for one another, that you may be healed. The effective, fervent prayer of a righteous man avails much (James 5:13, 15-16).

Do not assume God is ignoring you if you do not feel immediate results. He may require that you go through a learning process to truly become free of illness. He may even be ministering to others through your situation. Most of the healing that I have seen takes place as a natural progression as spiritual blocks are removed physically, mentally, and emotionally. For many of us, it takes time to learn how to do this.

Natural Healing According to God's Laws

Second, God's natural health principles promote the God-given ability of the body to heal itself at its optimum level. Poor health habits prevent this. If we choose to continue bad habits, we may reap from them what we sow. This is often why so many people resort to drastic and often invasive medical measures once their health begins to fail.

Challenge yourself to investigate and follow God's principles for abundant health. Natural health practitioners have long been assisting the body through natural principles of building, cleansing, healing, and energizing with the use of natural foods, herbs, essential oils, and therapeutic baths, to name just a few. People have reported amazing recoveries, such as reversed osteoporosis (deemed impossible not many years ago), improved eyesight, neutralized allergies, and dissolved tumors.

In the Bible, there is a story of a repentant king whose request for a health miracle is answered by God, combined with the application of natural health principles:

In those days Hezekiah was sick and near death. And Isaiah the prophet, the son of Amoz, went to him and said to him. "Thus says the LORD: 'Set your house in order, for you shall die, and not live.'" Then he turned his face toward the wall, and prayed to the LORD, saying, "Remember now, O LORD, I pray, how I have walked before You in truth and with a loyal heart, and have done what was good in Your sight." And Hezekiah wept bitterly. And it happened, before Isaiah had gone out into the middle court, that the word of the LORD came to him, saying, "Return and tell Hezekiah the leader of My people, 'Thus says the LORD, the God of David your father: "I have heard your prayer, I have seen your tears; surely I will heal you. On the third day you shall go up to the house of the LORD. And I will add to your days fifteen years. I will deliver you and this city from the hand of the king of Assyria; and I will defend this city for My own sake, and for the sake of My servant David." Then Isaiah said, "Take a lump of figs." So they took and laid it on the boil, and he recovered (2 Kings 20:1-7).

There are faith healers today who adamantly oppose herbs and other natural aids to health, choosing instead to rely only on God's hand in the matter. But as you see above, the king's health was restored through both spiritual and physical means. All true and good healing modalities are a gift from God. Explore them all and give thanks to God in the process.

HEALING PEARL:
SIN CAN BRING A CURSE UPON OUR HEALTH AND THE ENVIRONMENT

There is no soundness in my flesh because of Your anger, nor any health in my bones because of my sin. For my iniquities have gone over my head; like a heavy burden they are too heavy for me. My wounds are foul and festering because of my foolishness (Ps 38:3-5).

Were they ashamed when they had committed abomination? No! They were not at all ashamed, nor did they know how to blush. Therefore they shall fall among those who fall; in the time of their punishment they shall be cast down," says the LORD (Jer 8:12).
Is there no balm in Gilead, is there no physician there? Why, then is there no recovery for the health of the daughter of my people (Jer 8:22)?

Our total health and wellbeing does not solely depend on the knowledge of our physicians, but on the honor and respect we show our Creator. When our nation and its established systems tramples God's truths underfoot, we may risk reaping disastrous results.

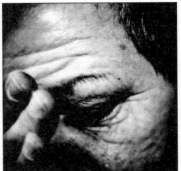

If you see sin in your country's modes and practices, do not partake in it. Be bold enough to speak out against any wrongdoing in hope that God will show His mercy.

(Zweettoth photo)

The earth is also defiled under its inhabitants, because they have transgressed the laws, changed the ordinance, broken the everlasting covenant. Therefore the curse has devoured the earth (Isa 24:5-6).

Note: "defiled" is sometimes translated "polluted."

Yes, this world is toxic with sin, but believers in Jesus Christ have been given the means to be victorious over sin and death.

Understanding Iniquities

Unfortunately mankind, in obeying selfish desires, can travel down the ill-fated path to destruction. The Bible calls these selfish desires iniquities, and they can be passed down through generations, affecting not only our health but the health of our children. It is imperative that we break their power in our lives so that we can be rid of them forever.

Primarily, iniquity denotes "not an action, but the character of an action" (Oehler), and is so distinguished from "sin" (chaTTa'th). Hence, we have the expression "the iniquity of my sin" (Ps 32:5).[10]

And the LORD passed before him and proclaimed, "The LORD, the LORD God, merciful and gracious, longsuffering, and abounding in goodness and truth, keeping mercy for thousands, forgiving iniquity and transgression and sin, by no means clearing the guilty, visiting the iniquity of the fathers upon the children and the children's children to the third and the fourth generation (Ex 34:6-7).

Unless we are extremely fortunate to have had a faithful, godly lineage, we all may carry the effects of iniquities.

Soon to follow is a sample prayer that may be used to renounce the negative patterns of any weaknesses of character, ethics, addictions, and morals that have passed down and affected us and our children. This is a prayer of love and restoration. It may be the most powerful prayer in this book. I see powerful changes in biofeedback data when this prayer alone is proclaimed aloud over one's entire being.

I believe that surfacing layers of inherited traumas and ancestral emotional debris are the biggest factors in some of the most stubborn health challenges.

A person may have to break these layers off in pieces as the body may not let it all go at once. This may be a protective mechanism of the body as the release of toxins appears to be a by-product of such prayers. Therefore, speak the prayer regularly and as tolerated when faced with serious challenges.

Consider praying aloud this prayer today, for yourself and over your young children. Encourage older children to read it or repeat it after you, assuring them that by doing so, they are not offending or rejecting you.

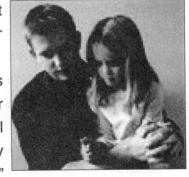

Personalize it by naming body parts from which you wish to see a particular release. I also verbally include "all cellular programming and energy patterns from any organ or body part" (say them by name) with serious or prolonged health challenges. I also like using anatomical charts for focused intention when I do these prayers. You may buy an anatomy book at a college bookstore, cut it up into body systems, and frame the systems into two large pictures for reference. Sometimes I have found it is important to name specific body parts to attain my goal of complete release.

RELEASING INIQUITIES PRAYER

Dear Heavenly Father, I acknowledge Your hand in my life and the purposes for which Christ came-- to truly set me free at every level of my being. Christ has offered to set me free so that I am free indeed. As a believer and your child, I now claim that promise!

I, therefore, in Jesus' name, cast off all unhealthy oppressions, curses, spiritual patterns, bindings, strongholds, addictions, compulsions, negative thinking patterns, unresolved emotions, physical ailments and genetic imperfections that cling to me from the iniquities of my male and female generational lineage as well as those from any step-parents or family back all generations to the beginning of time. I release them from all my cellular programming, memories, and energies.

Today, I claim Christ's sacrifice for my sins and total freedom from its effects on my character as provided by His death and resurrection and my belief in these. I rejoice in these Holy provisions. In the vacancies these releases create, I claim and place the development of Your mind and character within my own, with healthy physical, mental, emotional, and spiritual patterns as You originally intended for me. I am grateful for all blessings that my earthly parents and lineage have passed onto me. I forgive them for any mistakes as I ask forgiveness for my own. Thank you, Father, for Your loving mercy and forgiveness. I pray in Jesus' name. Amen.

Thankfully, iniquities need not master us any longer. In actively and verbally laying claim to Christ and His provision, we can rejoice because we have been bought for a price. Jesus' death paid the full ransom for sin, iniquity, and death.

> *Jesus answered them, "Most assuredly, I say to you, whoever commits sin is a slave of sin. Therefore if the Son makes you free, you shall be free indeed (John 8:34,36).*

Claiming the promise of this verse aloud and frequently over one's life and health is very powerful for healing. It is time to put a stop to negative generational cycles and addictive behaviors. We have been given the power to break those bonds when we lay claim to the promises of Jesus. Seek truth and promote godly change in your life. Do not participate in sinful behavior along with the world. Our offspring may reap the effects of our choices. Do what is good, true, and honorable, even if you must stand alone. God has called us to this standard, for His glory and for the good of the world. Reject passivity. Be a leader!

The Irish philosopher, Edmund Burke, once said that all that is needed for evil to triumph is for good people to do nothing.

HEALING PEARL:
GOD'S HEALTH PROVISIONS FOR OBEDIENCE TO HIS WORD

Children, obey your parents in the Lord, for this is right. "Honor your father and mother," which is the first commandment with promise: "that it may be well with you and you may live long on the earth" (Eph 6:1-3).

It is important to respect, honor, and speak well of our parents and grandparents. They give us many words of wisdom and guidance.

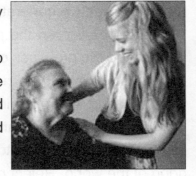

Following is a powerful verse to claim and personalize. Place it where you can see and say it daily to build your faith in the power of God's Word to affect your life!

But his delight is in the law of the LORD, and in His law he meditates day and night. He shall be like a tree planted by the rivers of water, that brings forth its fruit in its season, whose leaf also shall not wither; and whatever he does shall prosper (Ps 1:2-3).

Whatever I do shall prosper when following the Lord. What an amazing promise! Claim it aloud often as one of God's many gifts.

What if we reject or forget about God's teachings and help for our healing process? When we shut the door on God, He honors our choice to deal with our issues on our own terms.

Below is the tragic account of King Asa who did not appear to give consideration to God in his quest for healing.

> *Note that the acts of Asa, first and last, are indeed written in the book of the kings of Judah and Israel. And in the thirty-ninth year of his reign, Asa became diseased in his feet, and his malady was severe; yet in his disease he did not seek the LORD, but the physicians. So Asa rested with his fathers; he died in the forty-first year of his reign (2 Chron 16:11-13).*

It is not wrong to seek a physician's help, but it is a risk to leave God out of our healing regime. We should go to Him first in prayer. We are spiritual beings and it is wise to include a spiritual component in our healing.

The following verses relate a conversation between Jesus and Satan, during a moment when Jesus was extremely hungry after a prolonged fast. Here, it is stated clearly that remaining on the physical level alone is not sufficient:

> *Now when the tempter came to Him, he said, "If You are the Son of God, command that these stones become bread." But He answered and said, "It is written, 'Man shall not live by bread alone, but by every word that proceeds from the mouth of God'" (Matt 4:3-4).*

(Notice how Jesus counters Satan's temptations with Scriptures stated aloud--a great example for us.)

God's instructions often contain a condition, usually in the following words: "If you do...than I will do..." He grants us the ability to evaluate our choices. Every positive change reaps a positive effect.

Once you learn the principles of biblical health, it is a kindness to pass on these truths to receptive friends and family. Be patient and caring. Remember, it may have taken you some time to develop your health convictions. Relating them to others must be guided by love.

When Choosing Your Wellness Tools

There is a wide variety of often confusing choices in the field of traditional and alternative medicine. Where does one start?

Consider therapies that are non-invasive and health-promoting. Avoid the pitfall of adopting a negative view of any therapy or tool out of ignorance or arrogance. Some health practices, such as acupuncture and chiropractic, were first viewed with heavy skepticism by Western medicine, but are now widely accepted.

Do not be too quick to dismiss a healing modality because it resides outside of the framework of Western medicine. Doing so may rob you of valuable life-saving tools.

There are many healing modalities that God uses to accomplish His work. Whether or not they honor God depends on how they are used. Use discernment. Some practices are intertwined with philosophies that oppose God's teachings. It is worth considering the spiritual condition of the practitioner as it may color their entire approach to health and the tools he or she uses.

Science, with its limitations, has yet to completely understand how some assessments and therapies work in the realm of alternative and energetic medicine, such as acupuncture, muscle response testing, prayer, essential oils, far-infrared, gemstone therapy, therapeutic touch, flower essences, color therapy, sound therapy, zero point field energy therapy, various types of energetic frequency application, and more. There is a body of mounting and compelling evidence that suggest that these complementary methods are the next frontier of scientific discovery and research. Many are extremely valuable when used for alleviating certain health challenges. As non-invasive and health-supporting tools, they can glorify God in the process.

I am excited to believe that, in time, these forms of health care will become the mainstream of the future, as they address the body at its very energetic foundation. I believe we can all agree that the solution truly lies in getting to the root of the issue. Daily wonderful healings are taking place using remedies and principles not yet scientifically proven. When we come into agreement with God by believing in His words and power, and aligning our lives in obedience to Him, a door opens to miracles that we may never totally explain.

In conclusion, remaining solely at the level of physical health for our healing has its limitations. Many health challenges take a long time to resolve with physical help alone. A practitioner earnestly desiring to help others will do well to include God's principles of spiritual health that apply to mental and emotional states to enhance their clients' total health and well-being. Look for these practitioners in every branch of medicine.

CONCLUSION CHECKLIST

____In faith, I have started thanking my heavenly Father daily for the perfect healing that I seek in my quest to remove all obstacles to His blessings. I daily envision and proclaim what my healing will look like. I remember that everything is possible when God is in the picture.

____I have started buying more organic foods and using a vegetable and fruit wash (available in health stores) to remove any pesticides on produce that is not organic.

____I am becoming conscious of food quality. I read labels and ask questions. I am cooking "from scratch" more often. I avoid genetically modified foods, white sugar, high fructose corn syrup, trans-fats, bleached white flour, and other highly processed foods.

____I buy new healthy foods weekly, such as grapeseed oil and pomegranate juice. I utilize health food stores to broaden my horizons.

____I have considered and researched a quality water filtration system to provide pure water to my family and pets. (you can direct inquiries regarding our preferred systems to www.equippedtoheal.com)

____I avoid eating or drinking too much. I limit alcohol to twice weekly for my brain's sake. (Dr. Amen, brain expert, teaches that studies show that brain shrinkage occurs when consuming more than two cocktails weekly.)[12]

___I eat in a positive, relaxed atmosphere.

___I will evaluate natural medicine and explore the possibilities of herbs and essential oils for my health (www.equippedtoheal.com is a source of wholesale high quality herbs, oils, vitamins, and minerals. It features a search tool that helps locate the top three products for your health concern).

___I am willing to stand alone on what is right. I pray for my community, country, and world, and speak out against wrongs committed. I have begun to verbally release iniquities, trauma, and emotional baggage from my lineage.

___I persevere in my quest for health, seeking answers that bring me peace. I explore opportunities and suggestions that come my way. I realize God often works and speaks through people.

___I have recorded some of God's promises and keep them in my home and car for daily verbal affirmation. I am committed to aligning my whole being to God's truth.

___I gently and patiently share my pearls with those who are interested and refrain from judging those who are not.

___I am open-minded and do not take a negative view of new things just because I do not yet understand it. I realize that true healing is a gift from God.

___I look for health practitioners who employ mental, emotional, and spiritual truths along with healthy, non-harmful remedies when possible.

NOTES: _____

_____

_____

_____

_____

_____

_____

_____

_____

_____

_____

_____

_____

_____

_____

_____

_____

_____

_____

_____

_____

_____

_____

_____

_____

_____

_____

Part 2
Pearls of Mental Health

M ENTAL HEALTH: a state of mental peace, strength, and control where we evaluate, direct, and train our thoughts toward healthy thinking processes and decision making as God intended.

God loved us enough to give us the freedom to make our own decisions. He desires that we choose His best for us. Our choices play a major role in the course of our lives.

> I call heaven and earth as witnesses today against you, that I have set before you life and death, blessing and cursing; therefore choose life, that both you and your descendants may live; that you may love the LORD your God, that you may obey His voice, and that you may cling to Him, for He is your life and the length of your days [...] (Deut 30:19-20).

Our mind is a tool for survival. With choice, we are charged with the responsibility to logically and wisely analyze our situations. To do so, God gave us the ability to reason.

"Come now, and let us reason together," says the LORD [...] (Isa 1:18).

Thinking with logic and reason will give us the best, most accurate outcome while studying God's Word. It involves:

- Understanding the relevant facts.
- Understanding the sequence of events.
- Taking note of the time (present or past tense) and who is being addressed.
- Desiring a truthful conclusion.

This is a great foundation for the study of any topic. It is also our responsibility to think truthfully, positively, ethically, and morally. Challenge yourself to think for ten minutes weekly on how to better transform your life physically, mentally, emotionally, and spiritually. How might these transformations affect your job, your relationships, and your future?

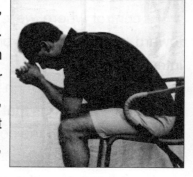

God likewise appeals to our minds for the transforming and maturing of our spirits. He challenges us to think and act on a higher plane that rises above our selfish desires.

And do not be conformed to this world, but be transformed by the renewing of your mind, that you may prove what is that good and acceptable and perfect will of God (Rom 12:2).

HEALING PEARL:
UNDERSTAND THE POWER OF YOUR THOUGHTS

Our beliefs direct our actions, which bring us either peace or misery. Following are some thoughts common to mankind that reflect the maturity of our thinking and beliefs. Can you predict the painful or healthy outcomes?

CHILDISH THINKING
    My parents, teachers, doctors, and pastors should be perfect.
ADULT MATURITY:
    When I allow others to have flaws as I do, I can forgive and honor them in their roles.

CHILDISH THINKING:
    My value depends on what others say or think.
ADULT MATURITY:
    God gave me self-worth as a part of His wondrous creation.

CHILDISH THINKING:
    People are always wounding me.
ADULT MATURITY:
    People wound others out of their own internal pain. How can I move forward in forgiving this person?

CHILDISH THINKING:
    If my life is perfect, then I will be content and happy.
ADULT MATURITY:
    Life involves both joy and suffering. True contentment arises out of spiritual maturity and a relationship with God.

CHILDISH THINKING:

If I am not perfect in my endeavors, I am a failure.

ADULT MATURITY:

God gives me grace in my failings as I rise again to my purpose.

> When I was a child, I spoke as a child, I understood as a child, I thought as a child; but when I became a man, I put away childish things (1 Cor 13:11).

> For as he thinks in his heart, so is he [...] (Prov 23:7).

Re-examine your core beliefs, especially if you are experiencing pain in your life. Are you still holding onto childish values? What you believe may not be the way things truly are. Re-examine everything.[13] It can be incredibly healing to put new endings on old stories.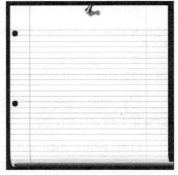

Boldly ask the Lord for maturity in thought and wisdom to make better choices, believing firmly that He will respond to your request. Commit to putting your trust in God's answers for your life. He is a master at making a door out of a wall. Stop riding the fence with unbelief, negative self-talk, and double-mindedness. It is time for change.

> Trust in the LORD with all your heart, and lean not on your own understanding; in all your ways acknowledge Him, and He shall direct your paths (Prov 3:5-6).

> If any of you lacks wisdom, let him ask of God, who gives

to all liberally and without reproach, and it will be given to him. But let him ask in faith, with no doubting, for he who doubts is like a wave of the sea driven and tossed by the wind. For let not that man suppose that he will receive anything from the Lord; he is a double-minded man, unstable in all his ways (James 1:5-8).

HEALING PEARL:
LIVE IN THE PRESENT

Take inventory of your thoughts. Are you making the past your present by allowing your thoughts to drift back into the land of mistakes, shame, and regrets? Are you allowing those who have hurt you to rent space in your head by obsessing over their past misdeeds? Are you fanning the flames of anger, vengeance, and oppression, lugging the past around like a cluster of heavy baggage? Consider the Apostle Paul's advice:

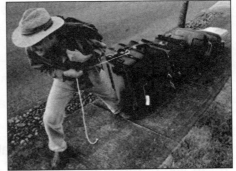

Brethren [...] one thing I do, forgetting those things which are behind and reaching forward to those things which are ahead, I press toward the goal for the prize of the upward call of God in Christ Jesus (Phil 3:13-14).

It is tough to move forward while looking backward. We are most successful in life when we learn the importance of releasing our baggage:

> *Then David left his baggage in the care of the baggage*
> *keeper, and ran to the battle line [...]*
> *(1 Sam 17:22, NASB®).*

David was smart. We can learn a valuable lesson from him. Fighting our battles in life is exhausting when our energies are divided. Christ has offered to take our baggage off our hands. Are you willing to give it to Him?

> *Come to Me, all you who labor and are heavy laden, and I*
> *will give you rest. Take My yoke upon you and learn from*
> *Me, for I am gentle and lowly in heart, and you will find rest*
> *for your souls. For My yoke is easy and My burden is light*
> *(Matt 11:28-30).*

It is time to inventory all patterns of stinkin' thinkin', negativity, blame, criticism, obsession, addiction, and anything else enslaving you.

When you are ready, verbally and boldly, in Jesus' name (for in His name is power), command all elements of your brain, thinking, and mental parts to release each unpleasant piece (by naming them), commanding these mountains out from your life, birth, gestation, and from any imprints of your male and female lineage.

By doing so, you may shed tears of relief and you may only feel like doing a little at a time. Each address may only break off five to ten percent of the bundles you are carrying, but it will always resolve something, whether you immediately realize it or not. The biggest mistake is to stop dealing with a reoccurring issue after a couple of sessions. You may need to repeat yourself several times, but these burdens will eventually lift. Other issues will periodically come to consciousness, letting you know they are next in line to be addressed.

After you release them, never leave a vacuum! Always put a healthy statement, affirmation, or Scripture in its place, such as the fruits of spiritual holiness and maturity mentioned in Galatians 5:22-23. For example:

> *"I replace this old baggage with healthy and positive thinking patterns filled with love, joy, peace, patience, kindness, goodness, faithfulness, gentleness, self-control, forgiveness, victory, and freedom!"*

This is one way to accomplish what the Word calls renewing your mind. Satan and his forces, as well as our own selfish desires, wage war with our minds through negative, self-defeating whispers which we must learn to discern and reject. Rebuke and resist all dark thoughts, whatever their origin, in the name of Jesus Christ. They are no match for you! Warn Satan that if he keeps bothering you, you will pray for ten extra people that day, and do it! Make it unprofitable and unpleasant for him to torment you.

There is no reason to fear any Satanic force on this earth. It has no claim over you unless you have let it in your life by either remaining apart from God or repeatedly ignoring your conscience and stepping out from God's protection. We can also invite darkness into our lives by dabbling in any branch of the occult. If you have given personal ground over to Satan and his wiles through sin, it is time to repent and verbally send him packing.

Therefore submit to God. Resist the devil and he will flee from you (James 4:7).

Claim aloud, with victory:

No weapon formed against me shall prosper!
(Isaiah 54:17).

This is one of the most powerful declarations in the Bible. It is given as a powerful protection by God for His people to claim. Consider applying it daily against Satan's attacks, disease, addictions, obsessions, and upsetting emotions.

The Importance of How We View Our Future

Do you over-think the potential problems that may occur in the future (and most of the time do not) with their tormenting fears? It is time to release the worries of tomorrow and replace them with the confidence that God will direct your future. His plans for you are good!

This healthy, productive way of thinking propels us toward growth, maturity, and peace. God wants us to be free of all fear, including fear of death. Trying to control every outcome in life is burdensome and impossible.

Now if God so clothes the grass of the field, which today is, and tomorrow is thrown into the oven, will He not much more clothe you, O you of little faith? Therefore do not worry, saying, 'What shall we eat?' or 'What shall we drink?' or 'What shall we wear?' For after all these things the Gentiles seek. For your heavenly Father knows that you need all these things. But seek first the kingdom of God and His righteousness, and all these things shall be added to you. Therefore do not worry about tomorrow, for tomorrow will worry about its own things. Sufficient for the day is its own trouble (Matt 6:30-34).

Please note the conditional promise surrounding "seek first the kingdom of God." Seeking one's own way instead of God's way may be one reason people and societies experience so much suffering in this world. When we seek first God's plans and instruction for us, He promises to meet our needs. We will be most at peace when we focus on the present and the confidence we have in God for the future.

Three hundred and sixty-five times in the Bible, God says, "Be not afraid..." That is one for each day if you need it.

HEALING PEARL:
GIVE CONSCIOUS, DAILY DIRECTION TO YOUR THOUGHTS BY GETTING RID OF A.N.T.S.

I enjoyed the A.N.T.S. exercise taught by Dr. Daniel Amen[14] based on four questions in *The Work* by Byron Katie Mitchell.[15] A.N.T.S are Automatic Negative Thoughts that consist of negative or worrisome things that could happen. We are encouraged to develop an internal "A.N.T. Eater" to eradicate them.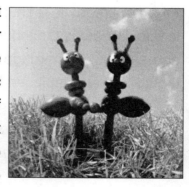

Thoughts can lie and accuse, especially if Satan throws them at us like darts. Examine and question A.N.T.S. Do not automatically believe them. Acknowledging and embodying a false thought can lead us to deviate from our true path and run into the ditch.

Here are *The Work's* four questions that address negative thoughts. They are worth memorizing:

1. Is it true?
2. Can you absolutely, positively know that it is true?
3. How do you react; what happens when you believe that thought?
4. Who would you be without that thought?

Many entertain incoming thoughts even though they may not be grounded in truth. When this happens, they may give rise to depression, fear, hopelessness, and more. If we choose not to believe a false thought, the ending is entirely different. Example:

"I am sixty-nine years old and single. No one will want to marry me."

I may at first believe this thought, but I cannot know for a fact it is true. Believing the thought may yield discouragement, despair, and sadness if marriage is a goal. How would I be if I let that thought go and replaced it with:

"I am sixty-nine years old and single, but someone out there would love to marry me!"

See how much better this feels! Now, how about erasing any projected negative endings you have been entertaining and write down your own positive ending to the open chapters in your life. Visualize and pray on these instead. You have a choice.

Do not choose that which leads to depression, fear, sorrow, and discouragement, or is contrary to God's teaching.

> *[...] casting down arguments and every high thing that exalts itself against the knowledge of God, bringing every thought into captivity to the obedience of Christ (2 Cor 10:5).*

> *Finally, brethren, whatever things are true, whatever things are noble, whatever things are just, whatever things are pure, whatever things are lovely, whatever things are of good report, if there is any virtue and if there is anything praiseworthy—meditate on these things (Phil 4:8).*

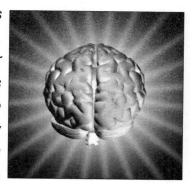

HEALING PEARL:
MENTAL STABILITY—SPEAK THE TRUTH

Our verbal speech and mental beliefs should be in harmony. We should speak the truth of our beliefs.

> *We having the same spirit of faith, according as it is written, I believed, and therefore have I spoken; we also believe, and therefore speak [...] (2 Cor 4:13).*

How many of us believe one thing yet speak the opposite? Some just stuff it all inside, never letting on if they disagree with what is popular in today's moral code or political correctness. Disagreement between our speech and beliefs is just one cause of stress and misalignment in our health.

Integrity is walking the walk and talking the talk. It is an important ingredient to physical health, mental stability, and peace. Keep in mind, I am not talking about brutal destructive honesty that leaves another shattered and distraught. We should always be honest and true to ourselves, but also be considerate, speaking the truth in love, kindness, and gentleness.

He who walks uprightly, and works righteousness, and speaks the truth in his heart [...] (Ps 15:2).

I tell the truth in Christ, I am not lying, my conscience also bearing me witness in the Holy Spirit (Rom 9:1).

The Insidious Snare of Lying

If we are honest, most of us at some time in our lives have been caught in a lie. If you are entangled in your own lies, it is time to take courage and, in humility, make things right.

You are snared by the words of your mouth; you are taken by the words of your mouth. So do this, my son, and deliver yourself; for you have come into the hand of your friend: Go and humble yourself; plead with your friend. Give no sleep to your eyes, nor slumber to your eyelids. Deliver yourself like a gazelle from the hand of the hunter, and like a bird from the hand of the fowler (Prov 6:2-5).

Admitting a lie is obviously embarrassing and humiliating. Be prudent when doing so. Think before speaking. Don't cast blame.

Even in the face of negative consequences, God desires us to speak the truth in a loving spirit with intent to build and repair relationships, not destroy them. It is important to our health on all levels that we are being true to God and ourselves. We have a conscience that bears witness to our mind and heart. When they are in agreement (and it may take prayer and meditation on the Word to determine this), we feel the most at peace about our decisions. Looking at yourself in the mirror at the end of the day should bring you pleasure, not pain.

HEALING PEARL:
THE MIRACULOUS POWER OF WORDS

With words alone, God created the world. God's words contain tremendous energy and power. Speaking God's Word aloud is powerful because His Holy Spirit infuses it.

For I am the LORD. I speak, and the word which I speak will come to pass (Ezek 12:25).

God's words make future events realities. When His words are sent out, the Scriptures states that they never return empty. When you share God's Word with others, it always have an impact, even if you cannot yet see it. Sharing it is never a waste of time. The Scriptures are a means by which we can receive eternal life and conquer sinful behaviors. The Psalmist agrees:

Your word I have hidden in my heart, that I might not sin against You (Ps 119:11)!

Because we are made in God's image, we have also been given a powerful gift within our words. Our words do not have the same authority or power as God's, but they are an amazing gift for a variety of reasons.

From a physics point of view, words are composed of frequencies and energies that can powerfully impact others, our environment, and especially anything comprised of water. That means our bodies, other people's bodies, food, and water are impacted by our words. To state it another way, what we say, think, and entertain mentally and emotionally can energetically imprint upon us, affecting our health. Since we are eighty percent water, positive, healthy words, thoughts, and emotions can be very healing to our bodies. The opposite is also true.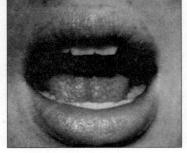

How do we apply this valuable information to our well-being? To begin, verbally and with conviction, speak a blessing of health and healing over and onto your food and beverages at meals. Be bold to command all contaminants and toxins to neutralize.

> *"In Jesus' name, may this food be blessed and nutritious*
> *to our bodies, and any contaminants and toxins be totally*
> *neutralized..."*

I can't stress enough how this changes the energetics of our foot for the better. If you take medications or receive vaccines, blood, or IVs, pray aloud over them (preferably while holding them) prior to their administration. I have even had food change in taste after doing this. Refer back to Judi's and Jon's prayers in Part One, if needed.

The energetic frequencies within words are a treatment in themselves—a marvelous gift from God. The last thing Satan wants you to discover is that God's provision has given you the power to heal yourself. Words are powerful healers, and destroyers, and should be used with caution and wisdom. The following verse is profound, with many incredible applications:

Death and life are in the power of the tongue, and those who love it will eat its fruit (Prov 18:21).

Again, we should always think before we speak. God desires that we speak truth and Scriptures into our lives, in trust and faith, thereby activating their full power to assist us.

Speak life and health daily to your body, mind, emotions, and spirit. Cast out all obstacles to these in Jesus' name, on a regular basis! The following verses contain a powerful lesson about verbally speaking to the obstacles that keep us from God's best.

For assuredly, I say to you, whoever says to this mountain, "Be removed and be cast into the sea," and does not doubt in his heart, but believes that those things he says will come to pass, he will have whatever he says. Therefore I say to you, whatever things you ask when you pray, believe that you receive them, and you will have them. And whenever you stand praying, if you have anything against anyone, forgive him, that your Father in heaven may also forgive you your trespasses. But if you do not forgive,

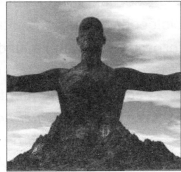

neither will your Father in heaven forgive your trespasses
(Mark 11:23-26).

What physical, emotional, mental, and spiritual mountains in your
life do you need to verbally remove? List them and command
them out. They are no match for you when armed with these
verses.

Be patient. Some obstacles may have numerous traumatic
and emotional patterns, whether or not we are aware of these.
They may not completely release all at once. I believe that a
proper time to release them is as we become aware of them.
Awareness of the entire issue may be a process that occurs over
time. Ask God to make them known in His proper timing.

Verbal speech has amazing power not only over our
physiology, but also our whole being. Evangelist Keith Moore
teaches that words are powerful when you say them aloud. Also,
faith grows from hearing yourself as well as others speak God's
truths.

Moore teaches that when we are speaking, we are doing (an
action). Speaking, then, is one way we can fulfill God's command
to be a doer of His Word. When we control our words, we can
control our bodies. Moore claims he has witnessed tumors shrink
with faith-filled words, sometimes immediately or over time.[16]

I see amazing evidence of the truth of these principles in
biofeedback sessions. For this reason, I suggest you make the
following command a fundamental part of your spiritual regime:

"I command all mountains in the way of my brain health,
liver health, mental health (... be creative!) to be broken
and released, and be replaced by God's perfect patterns
as He intended for my brain, liver, etc."

This is just one creative example. There are countless applications. (Something interesting that I have observed regularly is that people and pets yawn a lot as these stresses are verbally released. Yes, we can also pray these type of prayers over our pets with some pretty amazing results!)

Following are more examples of the amazing power of speech in action and its penetrating physical effects:

Pleasant words are like a honeycomb, sweetness to the soul and health to the bones (Prov 16:24).

The mouth of the righteous is a well of life [...] The tongue of the righteous is choice silver [...] The lips of the righteous feed many [...] (Prov 10:11, 20-21).

A wholesome tongue is a tree of life [...] (Prov 15:4).

My son, give attention to my words; incline your ear to my sayings. Do not let them depart from your eyes; keep them in the midst of your heart; for they are life to those who find them, and health to all their flesh (Prov 4:20-22).

HEALING PEARL:
NEITHER GIVE NOR ACCEPT VOODOO CURSES!

A "voodoo curse" is a tongue-in-cheek term we use in my office for anything said over another person that places a negative limitation on them.[17]

You may not think you are the terrifying character here, but you can surely sound like him with the words of your mouth.

Common voodoo curses include: "You can't...you won't... you'll never...you're so...you'll never get well...why can't you be more like... there is absolutely no cure...you only have six months to live!" Voodoo curses also include such proclamations as: "*Your* cancer...*your* diabetes...*your* arthritis, etc."

Do not admit ownership to a disease by calling it "mine." Experiencing disease is one thing, claiming it is another. The book, "Love, Medicine, and Miracles," by Bernie Siegel, documents the lives of supposedly doomed, sick people who defied their diagnosis in their return to health because they refused to accept negative pronouncements over their lives.[18]

If you believe a voodoo curse, it can have a tremendous power over you. Be aware that you may be more apt to adopt a voodoo curse when the person speaking it is an authoritative figure, such as a parent, doctor, teacher, pastor, or boss. Verbally negate or rebuke all curses immediately.

Oops, Did I Really Say That?

Have you ever spoken statements like these: "You're a drunk...you'll never change...you're always complaining...you'll never get well...you make so many wrong choices...you'll always be a loser." Or how about, "You eat fast food? Well, you deserve to be sick" or "You let your kids trick-or-treat in scary costumes? And you call yourself a Christian?"

God tells us not to curse, condemn, or pass a hateful judgment on another. Instead, lovingly correct, discipline, and uphold others if you feel them to be in error.

Also be careful that you do not hand down a sentence upon anyone, especially upon a weaker, less spiritually mature person who is in the process of learning. Trust that God is working in their lives.

Who are you to judge another's servant? To his own master he stands or falls. Indeed, he will be made to stand, for God is able to make him stand (Rom 14:4).

Our personal judgments can easily be made foolish by God's intervention. He has the power to lift up those we are judging and give them victory.

No Self-Curses!

Unfortunately, we can also curse ourselves, and creatively so. Following are some examples that should not be read aloud:

"I am such an idiot… beyond help… stupid…my body is so messed up…disgusting…fat… I will always be sick... I will never get well…I can't do that…I can't learn this…I can't be around cats…It is winter, I know I will get a cold soon…I can't stop smoking/drinking…Everything bad always happens to me…I am always in pain… I have no luck with men/women…I can never get ahead… I will never be successful, etc."

If you say these too many times, you will be right.

Even so the tongue is a little member and boasts great things. See how great a forest a little fire kindles! And the tongue is a fire, a world of iniquity. The tongue is so set among our members that it defiles the whole body, and sets on fire the course of nature […] (James 3:5-6).

With it we bless our God and Father, and with it we curse men, who have been made in the similitude of God. Out of the same mouth proceed blessing and cursing. My brethren, these things ought not to be so (James 3:9-10).

Whoever curses his father or his mother, his lamp will be put out in deep darkness (Prov 20:20).

Recall God's words regarding the power that our thinking, alone, has over our lives:

For as he thinks in his heart, so is he (Prov 23: 7).

Our words magnify this truth even further. We attract to ourselves what we believe, think, and say.[19] Decide today to stop hurling curses and harsh judgments at others and yourself. No matter how weak, sinful, or much of a mess others have made of their lives (or we have made of ours), our impatient judgments may prove inaccurate and foolish. God always reserves the right to intervene.

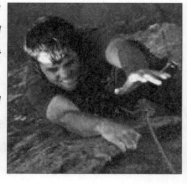

I waited patiently for the LORD; and He inclined to me, and heard my cry. He also brought me up out of a horrible pit, out of the miry clay, and set my feet upon a rock, and established my steps. He has put a new song in my mouth—Praise to our God [...] (Ps 40:1-3).

But I say to you that for every idle word men may speak, they will give account of it in the day of judgment. For by your words you will be justified, and by your words you will be condemned (Matt 12:36-37).

Have you been the recipient of a voodoo curse or harsh judgment?

Verbally renounce it! Break it! Speak blessings in its place. If you have pronounced voodoo curses over others, verbally repent and retract it. Speak blessings in its place towards the one you harmed. Apologize if needed.

Determine to clear out your inventory of childish thinking, negative outlooks, voodoo curses, and judgmental proclamations. Begin a new vocabulary today. Understand the incredible power of your words to alter the course of every aspect of your life.

HEALING PEARL:
LET THE WEAK SAY "I AM STRONG!"

Proclaim God's strength and truth into your life, especially in times of weakness. Proclamation is God's gift to His children. The Apostle Paul, having faith in God's strength, proclaimed, "I am strong!" when he felt weak, and he was strengthened. He trusted what God said and responded in kind:

And He said to me, "My grace is sufficient for you, for My strength is made perfect in weakness." Therefore most gladly I will rather boast in my infirmities, that the power of Christ may rest upon me. Therefore I take pleasure in infirmities, in reproaches, in needs, in persecutions, in distresses, for Christ's sake. For when I am weak, then I am strong (2 Cor 12:9-10).

He gives power to the weak, and to those who have no might He increases strength. Even the youths shall faint and be weary, and the young men shall utterly fall, but those who wait on the LORD shall renew their strength;

they shall mount up with wings like eagles, they shall run and not be weary, they shall walk and not faint (Isa 40:29-31).

Take these verses to heart. They act as powerful spiritual vitamins. With God's help, all things are possible. As you speak out your weakness, claim His might, power, and strength over every challenge on your journey. Proclaim "I am STRONG!" with full gusto and emotion, so as to reap its full power. Always think about what you are saying, and say it not once or twice, but many times. You may need to proclaim it aloud for one half hour daily if severe challenges are assaulting you. Be creative in your wording and application. How about:

"My kidneys are STRONG. My liver is STRONG. My immunity is STRONG. My lungs are STRONG. My digestion is STRONG. My ability to release all toxins from my cells is STRONG. My thyroid, adrenal glands, and sex glands are STRONG. My ability to conceive is STRONG!"

Do not limit yourself to the physical. Move into your mental, emotional and spiritual self. For example:

"My ability to be patient is STRONG. My ability to forgive is STRONG. My ability to focus on the positive is STRONG."

Now, choose to avoid all things that work against your strength. Evaluate movies, books, television, jobs, and friends that drain you of vitality on any level. Make positive changes that bring you health and wellness.

Be patient, waiting upon the Lord, for your full results.

Breaking an Addiction

Here is a paraphrase of an account by Pastor Keith Moore regarding a man who smoked for years and had tried many times, without success, to quit. Keith offered his help. The man assumed Keith would tell him, as did everyone else, to "just stop."

But Keith, full of surprises, gave him permission to smoke as he wished, with the condition that each time he either thought of a cigarette, bought a pack, lit up, or took a puff, he would proclaim aloud, "I am FREE from smoking!" The man agreed. After only six weeks, he excitedly reported that he had quit smoking.[20]

There is one who speaks like the piercings of a sword, but the tongue of the wise promotes health (Prov 12:18).

Use the power of your words for good. Resolve not to speak weakening words of unbelief and doubt. Dump your old negative vocabulary. Refuse to be a victim of life's circumstances. Stop asking "Why me?" Instead consider, "What amazing purpose will this serve in my life?" Be patient. As Christians, we wait upon the Lord. It is okay to not know all of the answers now.

And we know that all things work together for good to those who love God, to those who are the called according to His purpose (Rom 8:28).

Begin to strengthen yourself and others with words like, "I am (or am becoming) healthy and strong; things go well with me; I have faith in you; you will succeed."

Believe and do not doubt that God has good plans for you.

The way to change your life is to change your words. Do not say *"If* this good thing comes to pass." Say, in faith, *"When!"*

Of course, we must always leave room for God's will to supercede our own. If you have experienced the death of a dream or purpose you had for your life; please put an end to any despair. Believe with confidence that God has better plans in store for you than you may be able to imagine. Repeatedly claim this healing verse:

> *'For I know the plans that I have for you,' declares the LORD,' plans for welfare and not for calamity, to give you a future and a hope (Jer 29:11, NASB®).*

Adding mental alignment to your quest for health allows another big piece to fall into place. To align physically while neglecting your mental self is like taking two steps forward and one step backward. Dwell on the positives within your life. Speak health to yourself and others. Put a stop to unprofitable and unfruitful patterns or habits. Today is a great day to begin!

CONCLUSION CHECKLIST

___I am releasing childish thinking patterns that bring me pain and replacing them with mature adult thinking.

___I monitor my thoughts. I keep them focused on the present and on God's good plans for my future.

___I commit to God's guidance and best for me. I cease to be double-minded and unstable in my faith and actions.

___I commit to dumping my past baggage along with any of its tormenting influences. I refuse to allow it to be an obstacle to my healing.

___I am taking Automatic Negative Thoughts captive and giving them to the "A.N.T. Eater."

___I commit to guarding my mind against mental junk food on television, the news, in books, at the movies, and on the computer.

___I resolve when I pray about a subject to not afterward talk doubt and unbelief regarding the outcome, possibly negating my prayers due to a lack of faith.

___I resolve to stop talking negatively about others and myself. When someone complains about a person or a situation, I will not add to the negativity, but add positive comments only. I find the good in people and proclaim it. If I do not see the good, I pray for them, reminding myself that God made these people. He has plans for them to mature in goodness, just as my goodness is dependent on God's mercy in my life.

____I think before I speak. I am truthful in a gentle, loving way. I am a person of my word.

____I rely on the Lord's strength when I am weak. I verbally say, as many times as needed, "I am strong in the Lord!" I claim freedom in Christ from my weakness! I renounce my bad habits and addictions and speak out positive affirmations over all of them several times daily until I am victorious.

____I regularly speak out unwanted mental patterns and their effects from my mind, memory, focus centers, emotional centers, spinal cord, nerves, genetics, entire being, and any other areas of concern. I verbally replace them with positive, affirming thought patterns and Scriptures.

____I realize that the Bible is God's Will and Testament for His followers and that I, as a Christian, have a responsibility to lay claim to my inheritance. Just as I can be included in the will of a relative and yet not claim my inheritance, so can I neglect to claim the Scriptures that God has given for my healing. Claiming His Word aloud with proper motives is a powerful key to activation. I pray that everything I request is aligned with God's will for me, my family, and His ultimate purposes.

You lust and do not have. You murder and covet and cannot obtain. You fight and war. Yet you do not have because you do not ask. You ask and do not receive, because you ask amiss, that you may spend it on your pleasures (James 4:2-3).

NOTES: _____

Part 3
Pearls of Emotional Health

EMOTIONAL HEALTH: a state of stability involving love, grate-fulness, peace and joy, even in times of turmoil.

Easy to say, but challenging to do. It is a discipline that takes practice, and more practice, with a desire for personal growth. Emotional health is a by-product of correct decision-making and actions, as well as daily thankfulness for all of God's promises and blessings. It is accepting, with graciousness, that all pathways in life involve both suffering and joy that shape our character.

Emotions are an amazing and unique form of energy that prompts action. They have tremendous impact on our physiology for good or for bad, depending on how we manage them.

Unlike our bodies, emotions are not solid and visible, otherwise many of us would be tempted to schedule a surgical removal of our old painful hurts. Rather, they are a function of our

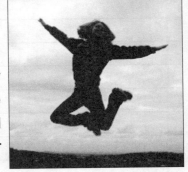

spirit, as evidenced by God Himself. We are made spiritually in His image. He is spirit and He expresses emotion.

When God expresses emotion, He follows it with action. Emotions are not negative unless poorly acted upon. When we manage them properly, we feel at ease. When we ignore the mature, spiritual action that should be the result of the emotional catalyst, we may feel uneasy, depressed, or miserable. Emotions are not the core of us, but a gift given to us from God. They are designed to be a tool for good.

Today, it is common for medical science to medicate what is often labeled "negative emotions." The same frequently occurs in natural medicine. As we study God's model, we may choose to redefine our approach. If emotions that bring suffering are processed wisely, the end result is peace.

As you learn to act upon your emotions properly, you may choose to re-evaluate with your doctor any medication you are taking, as the need may lessen. Adjusting medication without a doctor's help may be risky and is not recommended.

God Proclaims All of His Creation Good

So God created man in His own image; in the image of God He created him; male and female He created them. Then God saw everything that He had made, and indeed it was very good [...] (Gen 1:27,31).

"Everything" includes all of our God-given emotions. God's Word helps us understand how to express and deal with them properly.

The following is a helpful model for the classification of emotions, as inspired by Steven Horne, a well-respected author on natural and emotional health principles.[21] It is based on the concepts of *excessive*, *suppressed*, and *healthy emotional expression* (or put another way: *too much*, *too little*, or *just right (balanced)*.

Excessive Venting

When emotions continue to erupt excessively, there may be a wound within that has not healed properly. Some of us suffer from not knowing the true remedy for the wound. Others refuse, possibly subconsciously, to be healed.

Excess is apparent when emotions are recycled and vented for too long in hopes that someone or something external will somehow fix the issue. Physical organs become stressed. Friends and family, eager to assist at first, may become exhausted at the lack of resolution and, therefore, distance themselves.

Emotional Suppression

If we silently chew on and swallow our emotions, we risk them fusing with our psychology and physiology, resulting in depression, exhausted organs, and disease. Suppression is also a state of torment, as these emotions will not fail to issue periodic reminders that although they have been buried, they are certainly not dead.

Healthy Expression

This is where we pause to reflect and analyze our emotion. We avoid any immediate knee-jerk reactions that are destructive to our relationship with God and others. We express our emotions constructively and act upon their messages in a healthy manner. This is a by-product of spiritual growth. Potentially harmful emotions are resolved with reasonable action, the giving of any loose ends to the Lord for Him to handle, and a return to a state of peace.

Most of the emotions we struggle with fit into three primary groups. Please add any as you see fit.

The Anger Group
Anger, hatred, rage, accusation, aggression, rebellion, resentment, bitterness, unforgiveness, revenge, jealousy, betrayal, rejection, criticism, slander, stubbornness, bullying, impatience, and gossip.

The Sadness Group
Sadness, grief, despair, heartbreak, pain, abandonment, rejection, self-pity, depression, hopelessness, loneliness, possessiveness, neediness, selfishness, shame, and guilt.

The Fear-Worry Group
Fear, worry, anxiety, stress, tension, trauma, shock, addiction, paralysis, terror, timidity, insecurity, obsession, lying, greed, lust, and envy.

HEALING PEARL:
GOD'S RESOLUTIONS FOR ANGER

And the anger of the LORD burned against Uzzah [...]
(2 Sam 6:7, NASB®)

Then David's anger burned greatly against the man, and
he said to Nathan, "As the LORD lives, surely the man
who has done this deserves to die" (2 Sam 12:5, NASB®).

Common expressions for anger today include, "I saw red" or "He was so angry, he grew red in the face." Clearly we understand the heat and fire of anger.

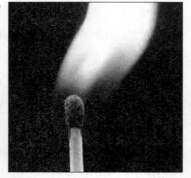

Anger commonly arises when we believe an unjust act has been committed or a boundary has been violated. Feeling angry is not wrong but what we do with it may be.

The knee-jerk response is to seek revenge or respond in kind. The healthy, spiritual response is to restore justice, dignity, and integrity to the situation without sinning. Many people in history have defended and achieved some of the noblest causes through the proper use of anger.

Physically, we may feel hot, irritated, and inflamed when holding onto anger. Inflammation is a foundational component of all disease. Symptoms may include joint pain, swelling, excess heat, high blood pressure, heart disturbances, excess adrenaline, insomnia, and hyperactivity of organs.

The Chinese medical model, the result of over two thousand years of observation, can help us understand how our emotional and physical parts interact. This model views the emotions and physical body as so completely entwined that they cannot be treated separately. Unprocessed emotions seem to reside in and affect specific body parts. Anger resides primarily in the liver.

The more anger, hatred, and rage we store, the more the liver may exhibit malfunction, toxic holdings, and inflammation.[22]

The Bible lends agreement that emotions reside in and impact our physical parts. Ecclesiastes 7:9 describes that fools allow anger to reside in their chests. God never intended for us to allow anger a home within our parts. Rather, we are to quickly diffuse the spark of anger with proper action before it turns into a raging inferno that threatens to destroy our health.

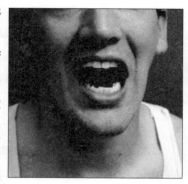

Although anger and its relatives can initially affect the liver and chest, they may store throughout the body if we let them progressively mount. Give top consideration to any physical part that is inflamed, painful, hyperactive or swollen, when speaking the freeing prayers of emotional release that are at the end of this section.

Excessive Venting

The impulsive venting of hateful words and actions usually comes back to bite us. Sometimes it erupts suddenly when someone unintentionally treads upon one of our unhealed wounds. Impulsive venting often leaves us mired in shame and regret.

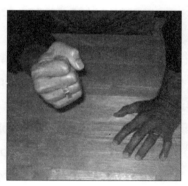

Those who excessively vent earn the reputation of being *hot-tempered*. The wounded party may respond in kind. Relationships may be harmed and the repair process unpleasant. When possible, avoid associations with chronically-angry people.

Make no friendship with an angry man, and with a furious man do not go, lest you learn his ways and set a snare for your soul (Prov 22:24-25).

Wrath is cruel and anger is a torrent, but who is able to

stand before jealousy (Prov 27:4)?

An angry man stirs up strife, and a furious man abounds in transgression (Prov 29:22).

Hating Others May Be A Sign that YOU Have Acted Inappropriately

In 2 Samuel, there is an interesting account of the emotionally volatile Amnon, son of King David, who is consumed by his sexual obsession with his half-sister, Tamar.

After this Absalom the son of David had a lovely sister, whose name was Tamar; and Amnon the son of David loved her. Amnon was so distressed over his sister Tamar that he became sick; for she was a virgin. And it was improper for Amnon to do anything to her (2 Sam 13:1-2).

Allowing his emotional impulses to rule, Amnon deceptively pretended to be bedridden and hungry.

Now when she had brought them to him to eat, he took hold of her and said to her, "Come, lie with me, my sister." And she answered him, "No, my brother, do not force me, for no such thing should be done in Israel. Do not do this disgraceful thing! And I, where could I take my shame? And as for you, you would be like one of the fools in Israel. Now therefore, please speak to the king; for he will not withhold me from you." However, he would not heed her voice; and being stronger than she, he forced her and lay with her. Then Amnon hated her exceedingly, so that the hatred with which he hated her was greater than the love with which he had loved her. And Amnon said to her, "Arise, be gone!" (2 Sam 13:11-15).

This account portrays some important principles. First, notice that Amnon was offered the remedy for what he should do to diffuse his frustrations, but he chose to ignore it. Instead, he followed his first impulse, which soon gave way to the misdirected fire of hatred. For the grand finale, Amnon deflects the hatred of his act away from himself and toward an innocent party.

We learn here that it is important to be honest with ourselves when identifying the root of any hatred. Is the hatred the result of another person's actions, or our own? With whom does the issue truly lie?

When we offend another person, even if it is a secret offense such as gossiping or breaking a rule, we may project the beginning feelings of self-hatred and contempt onto them, avoiding the true weakness within ourselves.

Following are a couple of examples as food for thought and discussion. Where do you think the true root of the anger lies?

1. An unruly teen treats his or her parents with contempt and disrespect when the bewildered parent simply tried to have a normal conversation. *"Where did that reaction come from?"* the parent wonders. Unbeknownst to the parent, the teen has made several bad choices and kept them secret so as to avoid disapproval or punishment.
2. A person with a strong personality is usually pressing to have her plans dominate those of a passive friend. Even though the friend may not enjoy the activity, he or she says little and often complies. With rising discontent, the passive friend begins to

vent by gossiping and complaining to others.

How may these principles about anger apply to you and your interactions? Continually venting hatred and anger may be the way you try to heal, but it only makes matters worse.

Ask yourself, "What hurts me so deeply that I am trying to heal by hurting others?"

Those who have not submitted to God's will for their total health may have many emotional challenges, having adapted to surviving on poorly managed emotions. It is challenging for spiritual messages to reach those whose have fused their psychology and physiology with hatred, victimization, and revenge. If someone chooses to remain at this level, he or she is, in essence, choosing to subsist on spiritual junk food. This can result in resistance to change as well as a foundation for disease. We know we have gone too far in our anger when even our bodies are begging us to change!

Anger Suppression

If we internalize our anger, we risk resentment, bitterness, hatred, and depression entrenching deeply into our physiology. Gossip and passive aggression may be the results of avoiding the root issue. Our spirits repeatedly bring the problem to our conscious mind in the hopes that we will deal with it properly. Sadly, in ignorance, stubbornness, or both, we often choose to chew on it all over again and stuff it back down. Following is an example of the suppression then explosion of anger, and its tragic result.

Now Abel was a keeper of sheep, but Cain was a tiller of the ground. And in the process of time it came to pass that Cain brought an offering of the fruit of the ground to the

LORD. Abel also brought of the firstborn of his flock and
of their fat. And the LORD respected Abel and his offering,
but He did not respect Cain and his offering. And Cain was
very angry, and his countenance fell (Gen 4:2-5).

His countenance has to do with his appearance and emotional state. Cain was possibly inclined to be stingy, which may have been God's issue with him in the first place. "Fat" portions may have had the connotation of abundance and generosity. The Bible records God's acceptance of plant offerings when offered according to His guidelines.

Then the LORD said to Cain, "Why are you angry? And
why has your countenance fallen? "If you do well, will not
your countenance be lifted up? And if you do not do well,
sin is crouching at the door; and its desire is for you, but
you must master it." And Cain told Abel his brother. And it
came about when they were in the field, that Cain rose up
against Abel his brother and killed him
(Gen 4:6-8, NASB®).

God informs Cain that it is up to him to master his impulses. If he does not, he will face some certain consequences. Cain listens, then makes his decision. He opts to follow his initial impulses in the heat of his intense emotion. The same is often true for us. Instead of mastering our emotions, we gratify them.

On a Side Note: The Importance of Mastering Sin

When we do not take our thoughts captive and evaluate them before assimilating them into our beliefs and actions, we risk giving ground to evil and becoming a vehicle for Satan's temptations and dark expressions. Our true war is not with mankind, but with the sin and evil that so easily entangles us.

Woe to the inhabitants of the earth and the sea! For the devil has come down to you, having great wrath, because he knows that he has a short time (Rev 12:12).

For we do not wrestle against flesh and blood, but against principalities, against powers, against the rulers of the darkness of this age, against spiritual hosts of wickedness in the heavenly places (Eph 6:12).

Are you entertaining thoughts and ideas that may belong to this realm? The following verses list a few examples of how people can invite Satan into their lives to exact his corruption:

There shall not be found among you anyone who makes his son or his daughter pass through the fire, or one who practices witchcraft, or a soothsayer, or one who interprets omens, or a sorcerer, or one who conjures spells, or a medium, or a spiritist, or one who calls up the dead. For all who do these things are an abomination to the LORD, and because of these abominations the LORD your God drives them out from before you. You shall be blameless before the LORD your God (Deut 18:10-13).

Note: Soothsaying can be translated "divination"--the attempt to contact a supernatural entity for information.

The Israelites received these exhortation after they had drifted away from the Lord and his teachings and sunk into a moral low that included sacrificing their children in fire.

How are we to guard ourselves against Satan's influences and deceptions?

Finally, my brethren, be strong in the Lord and in the power of His might. Put on the whole armor of God, that you may be able to stand against the wiles of the devil (Eph 6:10-11).

Stand therefore, having girded your waist with truth, having put on the breastplate of righteousness, and having shod your feet with the preparation of the gospel of peace; above all, taking the shield of faith with which you will be able to quench all the fiery darts of the wicked one. And take the helmet of salvation, and the sword of the Spirit, which is the word of God; praying always with all prayer and supplication in the Spirit, being watchful to this end with all perseverance and supplication for all the saints (Eph 6:14-18).

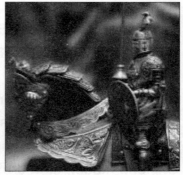

Satan is cunning in his acts and influence. He is always looking to undermine any vulnerable spots in our armor. Learn discernment through the study of God's Word. Guard your heart and mind. Take courage and know that God wants you to be free.

Anger's Relative: Gossip

Gossip is a destructive form of retaliation that is often rooted in pride, suppressed anger, fear of confrontation, and spiritual immaturity.

The words of a talebearer are as wounds, and they go down into the innermost parts of the belly (Prov 18:8, KJV).

If irritations in relationships are not resolved properly, we may feel tempted to act aggressively and gossip. If I catch myself gossiping, it becomes clear to me that I have not handled the conflict. If I resolve the conflict in a proper manner, there is no desire to gossip.

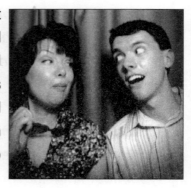

HEALING PEARL:
GOD'S ANTIDOTE FOR BITTERNESS

Bitterness is a state of torment that arises when strong emotions begin to fester. Bitterness affects our energy and may easily lead to physical and emotional depressions and imbalance. In our Chinese model, stored bitterness and resentment reside mainly in the gallbladder, but Biblically, there are also references to its storage in the bones where important aspects of our immunity lie.

It may be imperative to release all old stored unforgiveness toward men, women, children, God, one's family tree, society, and oneself. Consider commanding out, in Jesus' name, all mountains of resentment and bitterness, especially from the liver, gallbladder, immunity, bone marrow, all joints, bones, and cells.

In the New Testament, Simon the sorcerer is described as having the "gall of bitterness," which acts as an obstacle to his spiritual growth.

But Peter said to him, "Your money perish with you, because you thought that the gift of God could be purchased with money! You have neither part nor portion in this matter, for your heart is not right in the sight of God. Repent therefore of this your wickedness, and pray God if perhaps the thought of your heart may be forgiven you. For I see that you are poisoned by bitterness and bound by iniquity." Then Simon answered and said, "Pray to the Lord for me, that none of the things which you have spoken may come upon me" (Acts 8:20-24).

Bitterness, here, is described as a poison. Some of us are so concerned about releasing toxic buildup from our bodies, while perhaps neglecting an emotional poison that is even more insidious.

It is interesting to note that with all of Simon's problems, he is extremely alert to the incredible power of words.

Throughout Scripture, the bondage and misery that characterizes bitterness is coupled with many other issues, such as hostility, poisonous 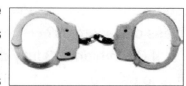 thought processes, grief, anguish, self-hatred, suicidal thoughts, joylessness, injustice, hardship, affliction, cursing, and falling captive to sin.

The following verses list a few humbling actions that act to soften or neutralize anger and bitterness.

Let all bitterness, wrath, anger, clamor, and evil speaking be put away from you, with all malice. And be kind to one another, tenderhearted, forgiving one another, just as God in Christ forgave you (Eph 4:31-32).

Pursue peace with all people, and holiness, without which no one will see the Lord: looking diligently lest anyone fall short of the grace of God; lest any root of bitterness springing up cause trouble, and by this many become defiled (Heb 12:14-15).

In all cases of anger and its relatives, God asks us to take actions that may feel unnatural and yet are the spiritual antidotes for our feelings of trouble and injustice.

"But I say to you who hear: Love your enemies, do good to those who hate you, bless those who curse you, and pray for those who spitefully use you (Luke 6:27-28).

Bless those who persecute you; bless and do not curse (Rom 12:1).

The word "bless" means "to speak well of." How do we love and bless our enemies?

I Corinthians 13 fully defines what love is (an action) and how it is to be expressed to others:

Though I speak with the tongues of men and of angels, but have not love, I have become a sounding brass or a clanging cymbal. And though I have the gift of prophecy, and understand all mysteries and all knowledge, and though I have all faith, so that I could remove mountains, but have not love, I am nothing. And though I bestow all my goods to feed the poor, and though I give my body to be burned, but have not love, it profits me nothing. Love suffers long and is kind; love does not envy; love does not parade itself, is not puffed up; does not behave rudely, does not seek its own, is not provoked, thinks no evil; does not rejoice in iniquity, but rejoices in the truth; bears all things, believes all things, hopes all things, endures all things. Love never fails (I Cor 13:1-8).

If you hold a postcard close enough to your face, it can obscure your

view of the Grand Canyon! Similarly, holding onto a wrong in the foremost of your mind can keep you from seeing all of your blessings. Please do not toy with bitterness. Refuse to carry the torment any longer. Give it to the Lord aloud until it is gone. Forgive in person, or go into your closet and do it.

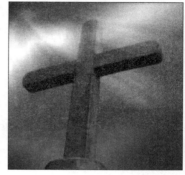

Change your actions toward the one who has been the target of your bitterness. Do something nice for them. Enjoy their surprise and your inner healing.

Dealing with Hatred

Hatred or intense anger is destructive when targeted against others, but positive when targeted against injustice with the intent to end it.

When we hate the evil deeds of others, we should respond with spiritually sound speech and actions. If we find ourselves hating someone, then we need to shift our hatred onto the wrong committed. Below is an example of hatred properly channeled, not toward the person, but toward the wrongful deed:

But this you have, that you hate the deeds of the Nicolaitans, which I also hate (Rev 2:6).

Sometimes we may hate our or someone else's spiritual immaturity and weakness. The Apostle Paul stated his inner struggles between good and evil.

> *For I know that in me (that is, in my flesh) nothing good dwells; for to will is present with me, but how to perform what is good I do not find. For the good that I will to do, I do not do; but the evil I will not to do, that I practice. Now if I do what I will not to do, it is no longer I who do it, but sin that dwells in me (Rom 7:18-20).*

> *O wretched man that I am! Who will deliver me from this body of death? I thank God—through Jesus Christ our Lord (Rom 7:24-25)!*

The flesh refers to our natural, impulsive, and often immature responses that we must learn to control through spiritual teaching and growth. Living in the flesh is also descriptive of a life lived apart from Christ. Without God's remedy for sin, it is all too easy to develop hatred of self and others. Paul expresses the wretchedness of his condition as well as his gratefulness for God's provisions by which he may have victory over his selfish desires.

We all wrestle with evil, temptation, and sin. By seeing sin as an affliction rather than an inherent character trait, we are better able to have love and compassion for people and help them.

The Healthy Expression of Anger

God, in His love for us, conveys a sense of control and urgency in dealing with these strong emotions so that we do not give Satan opportunity.

So then, my beloved brethren, let every man be swift to hear, slow to speak, slow to wrath (James 1:19).

Be angry, and do not sin: do not let the sun go down on your wrath, nor give place to the devil (Eph 4:26-27).

Regardless of who is at fault, we are not to wait for the other person to make things right.

Therefore if you bring your gift to the altar, and there remember that your brother has something against you, leave your gift there before the altar, and go your way. First be reconciled to your brother, and then come and offer your gift (Matt 5:23-24).

The best approach to reconciliation is humbly apologizing, asking forgiveness for your part of the offense (even if you do not see your offense), and resist speaking blame (this is the most crucial part). Your grace, spiritual maturity, and gentleness in the matter will play a part in softening the heart of the other, and promoting a healthy resolution. Ideally, both parties find forgiveness and respect. If this does not occur, however, we can still be at peace by accepting that we did everything we could to heal the situation.

If circumstances prevent resolution, then I suggest letting it go verbally:

I forgive Mom, Dad, my co-worker, etc. I release it. I forgive because I have been forgiven. I release all mountains of resentment, unforgiveness, and injustice from anywhere it has stored in my being. I give it to the Lord to take, and I replace it with mercy, compassion, and love.

The root word of "forgive" is *to* "exhale." Take a deep breath and let it all out. You may need to do this several times over a period of time. More will release each time. You will know you are done when you no longer feel the sting of the event and can simply focus on the lesson learned.

Feeling the Desire for Revenge?

Forgiving is not excusing or justifying the other person's behavior. Forgiving frees us from bearing the stress of this heavy baggage.

Verbally forgive and give your burden and any feelings of injustice to God. God willingly takes our baggage so that we may heal. He comforts us with the promise to someday avenge all injustice, whether now or in the life to come.

For rulers are not a terror to good works, but to evil. Do you want to be unafraid of the authority? Do what is good, and you will have praise from the same. For he is God's minister to you for good. But if you do evil, be afraid; for he does not bear the sword in vain; for he is God's minister, an avenger to execute wrath on him who practices evil (Rom 13:3-4).

Beloved, do not avenge yourselves, but rather give place to wrath; for it is written, "Vengeance is Mine, I will repay," says the Lord (Rom 12:19-20).

Rulers are the legal authorities of the 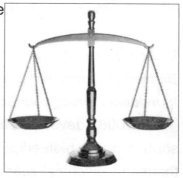 approval to exact justice on wrongdoers. However, if the legal system fails us, God takes justice into His own hands and executes His wrath upon the perpetrator in His own perfect timing. With God in control, we are to let go of any desire to avenge ourselves. Christians are encouraged scripturally to resolve disputes with fellow Christians, with the church's guidance if needed, so as to not enter the legal system. It is a sad day when two Christians go to court against each other.

Anger, hatred, and their relatives are complex and intense emotions. They work together for good if acted upon properly. It is important to resolve feelings of anger in a timely manner by turning them into a positive action. Act on what you can change, and verbally let go of what you cannot.

Strife in this world should not determine your level of emotional health and joy, or else you will forever be on an emotional roller coaster. Reside always within the intimacy and grace of our loving God. See yourself in the refuge of His perfect love, even in times of turmoil, with His arms lovingly wrapped around you. Determine to stay in the embrace of that peace at all times, even when chaos swirls around you. I often pause and say to myself, "I can deal with this difficult challenge while resolving to stay at peace internally, or I can deal with it with anger, anxiety, grief, and stress. Which is better?"

Decide to show love to others even when it is not returned. Love of this kind does not have to do with liking the person or having warm feelings. It has to do with treating others as you would like to be treated. We can and should see the good in others as they are all creations of God.

Biofeedback Study:

Biofeedback results from releasing anger and similar emotions in individuals through verbal prayer.

In 2008, I developed a small, informal study using an extremely sophisticated biofeedback system that measures over eight thousand electrical readings in the human body. It uses these readings to treat stress with energetic frequencies. The purpose is to assist the body in healing itself of its stressful patterns. I observed an interesting and exciting trend in twenty volunteers.

First, I recorded non-diagnostic electrical scores in the following categories.

1. Voltage (an electrical reading often improved by assisting healthy adrenal function).
2. Amperage (an electrical reading often improved by assisting healthy brain function).
3. Resistance (an electrical reading often improved with healthy cleansing and immune support).
4. Hydration (an electrical reading often improved with healthy water absorption into the cells).
5. Oxygenation (an electrical reading often improved with healthy oxygenation of the cells).

I also took note of organ stress profiles and general computer-suggested therapies.

Without using any computer-suggested therapies, I asked all volunteers to verbally recite the freedom prayer regarding the anger group of emotions.

After refreshing the computer screen, the general computer-suggested therapies disappeared or were reduced, sometimes dramatically.

Client scores, as a group, improved by the following percentages: Three by twelve percent, three by fourteen percent, three by sixteen percent, one by eighteen percent, one by twenty percent, three by twenty two percent, three by twenty four percent, two by twenty six percent and one by twenty eight percent!

Amazing results for just a few minutes of work! I continue to see similar results in all of my clients who consent to doing the prayers.

The Conclusion

Working at the emotional level is an inexpensive and powerful form of health care. There is mounting evidence that it alters our body chemistry, the way we detoxify, the energy flow of the body, and the ability to fight off invaders and abnormal cells. With regular attention, emotional work may literally save our lives.

A mighty God has given us the ability to heal ourselves by speaking and claiming the Word and its principles over our lives. God has already given us the tools. Let's lay claim to them.

Praise Him who makes healing not a matter of riches or means, but of trust, faith, and obedience!

CONCLUSION CHECKLIST

____I have made a list of the inflaming substances that I am exposed to in excess, such as alcohol, coffee, cigarettes, pesticides, food additives, drugs, chemical cleansers, etc. I realize that if these accumulate in my body, especially in my liver, I may feel irritated emotionally, possibly without further external causes.

____I have taken inventory of the anger family. Who are the objects of my heated emotions? If others are encroaching upon my boundaries and taking advantage of me, I am deciding how I can stand up for myself gently, firmly, and respectfully. I will treat others as I wish to be treated.

____I will be more aware of any issues of anger that arise, and I commit to resolving them that day when possible.

____I commit to expressing anger in a non-destructive way, letting go of all personal desires for vengeance apart from the action of legal authorities. I place all outcomes in God's hands.

____I will take note of injustices that spark my anger. How can I channel my anger into actions that solicit God's approval and make a difference in my neighborhood, community, and world?

____I have made a list of those I need to forgive. I choose to see their wrongdoing as something that is not a true part of who they are but a manifestation of their wounds. I realize that forgiving verbally is good for me, my relationship with God, and the one I forgive.

___I will keep any bitterness in perspective and not allow it to obscure my view of the blessings in my life. I will work to let go of any bitterness.

___What I send out comes back to me. I reap what I sow. What am I reaping that I hate? What can I do about it?

___I commit to monitoring any desire to gossip. I will talk directly to the party with whom I am feeling critical, with the goal of resolving the conflicts the day they occur. I will be self-controlled and gentle. I will learn to persuade with reason and love.

___I have meditated on whether I have done something wrong to an innocent party and find myself wrongfully hating them. I have been honest about where the true issue lies. I know it is not too late to change my behavior and attitude. I will ask forgiveness from God and others when needed so as to restore proper relationships. I will also forgive myself.

NOTES: _____

_____

_____

_____

_____

_____

_____

_____

_____

_____

_____

_____

_____

_____

_____

_____

_____

_____

_____

_____

_____

_____

_____

_____

_____

_____

_____

_____

_____

_____

VERBAL FREEDOM PRAYER FROM ANGER

I am determined to move on and release all mountains in my life. In Jesus' name, I command all mountains of anger, rage, hatred, bitterness, accusation, blame, resentment, unforgiveness, rebelliousness, and all conflicts, traumas or spiritual oppression to which these are connected, to release completely from wherever they have attached to my being: my genetics, energies, body, thinking patterns, emotional centers, soul, and spirit.

I especially command all forms of anger from all energetic and cellular programming of my head, brain, neck, chest, central zone, pelvic zone, legs, immunity, bones and bone marrow, all spinal parts, liver, gallbladder, intestines, heart, lungs, breasts, joints, lymph, veins, arteries, fat, and any areas of inflammation, swelling, pain, and abnormal tissues. I am done with them and send them to the feet of Jesus.

I forgive all men, women, and children that come to mind (name them if names come to mind) and all those that do not come to mind. I forgive myself of all my errors. I release any blame toward God.

I release all forms of anger and their offspring from any attachment to my life, birth, gestation, and any that have been imprinted through genetics, and all iniquities from my mother's and father's family trees, back through the generations to the beginning of time. I ask forgiveness for holding onto any of these.

Now in these vacancies, I claim healthy physical, mental, emotional, and spiritual patterns as God intended. I accept into my being - love, joy, peace, patience, kindness, goodness, faithfulness, gentleness, self-control, mercy and compassion toward others, and forgiveness as I have been forgiven by my Father in heaven.

Thank you, Lord! Amen.

Consider speaking this prayer slowly with intent and visualization, and in conjunction with the two forthcoming prayers in this section and the Trauma Prayer in Appendix IV. Consider this every one to two weeks to evict stored emotional layers as they become ready to release. You may also wish to release any specific memories connected to them. It can take some weeks or months to completely untangle all the emotions and traumas from certain life events. Persevere!

HEALING PEARL:
GOD'S RESOLUTIONS FOR SORROW, GRIEF, AND HEARTBREAK

All forms of loss, especially death, contribute heavily to these distressing emotions. Though painful, death teaches us the incredible value of life. Sorrowful emotions begin the healthy process of learning to let go of everything that is temporary. They remind us to see each day as a gift, and that ultimately all sorrows will be resolved through God's promise of eternal life.

And God will wipe away every tear from their eyes; there shall be no more death, nor sorrow, nor crying. There shall be no more pain, for the former things have passed away." Then He who sat on the throne said, "Behold, I make all things new." And He said to me, "Write, for these words are true and faithful" (Rev 21:4-5).

Sorrow stresses our bodies and gives us "the blues." When sorrow resides in us, we often feel sluggish and unmotivated, sometimes to the point of exhaustion. We feel sorrow in our chest and call it heartbreak. People often clutch their chest when receiving sorrowful news. Hearts may literally ache from grief.

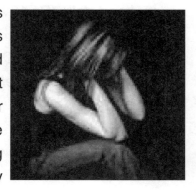

Sorrow in the Chinese Model (see Appendix III) predominantly resides in the chest, especially the lungs, but it can also invade other areas if prolonged. Scripturally, sorrow can store in the heart and eyes.

Symptoms may include heart challenges, shallow breathing, sighing, poor posture, shoulder tightness, arm numbness, diaphragm tension, lung conditions that may include pain or weakness, feelings of coldness, congestion, depression, poor circulation, and fatigue.

Excessive Venting

The Bible justifies a period of grief and mourning. People then (and in some countries today) were very expressive of their grief. They tore their clothing, dressed in mourning clothes, and wept bitterly to release their sorrow. The book of Lamentations has many examples of this. Our current funeral services make allowance for mourning with others for a few days, but, for some, a few days is not enough. The imbalance of excessive sorrow occurs when sorrow becomes prolonged with no goal of resolution.

How long shall I take counsel in my soul, having sorrow in my heart daily (Ps 13:2)?

Have mercy on me, O LORD, for I am in trouble; my eye wastes away with grief, yes, my soul and my body (Ps 31:9)!

[...] I have great sorrow and continual grief in my heart (Rm 9:2).

Unresolved sorrow brings misery to both body and spirit. It may lead to exhaustion and even death. This seems to be especially true in the elderly.

Then He said to them, "My soul is exceedingly sorrowful, even to death. Stay here and watch with Me" (Matt 26:38).

When He rose up from prayer, and had come to His disciples, He found them sleeping from sorrow (Luke 22:45).

Excessive, unrelenting sorrow can paralyze one's life from moving forward. It creates the potential for complaining, pessimism, self-pity, depression, apathy, extreme fatigue, and disease. As with the unresolved venting of anger, friends and acquaintances who are usually eager to offer comfort at first, may begin to withdraw from the situation.

The venting of emotions that resist resolution can often form a contaminating cloud that has a tendency to cling to and invade others who have their own vulnerabilities.

Suppressed Sorrow

We may unknowingly contribute to suppressed sorrow with words like, "Don't cry, that's for sissies"..."Stop crying before I spank you!"..."Why don't you toughen up?"..."Men don't cry!" Suppressed sorrow may manifest in the avoidance of intimacy, social functions, and other areas where there is the potential for new heartache to occur.

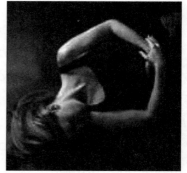

Some choose to reside in their heads so as to avoid contact with the feelings of their heart. Others become mired in pessimism and self-centered actions, which may lead to depressive and suicidal thoughts.

Symptoms of depression, poor energy, exhaustion, chronic chest complaints, shoulder slumping, eye imbalances, and poor immunity may manifest.

Guilt, shame, and condemnation of self, others, or God can entwine with grief, and may include tormenting thoughts: "I, others, or God could have…should have." If these feelings remain unresolved, they may pollute our conscience and shipwreck our faith.

This charge I commit to you, son Timothy…having faith and a good conscience, which some having rejected, concerning the faith have suffered shipwreck
(I Tim 1:18-19).

To cleanse our conscience of guilt or shame connected to unresolved sorrows, we may need to forgive ourselves, others, society, and God. Verbally doing this in person or alone in a quiet place may be tremendously more powerful and effective than doing it silently.

When we first confess belief in Christ's ability to redeem our lives, God provides a way for us have a good conscience towards Him:

The like figure whereunto even baptism doth also now save us (not the putting away of the filth of the flesh, but the answer of a good conscience toward God
(1 Pet 3:2, KJV).

Immersion in water symbolizes a burial of our old life and all of its mistakes. Through it and afterward, we are continually granted God's forgiveness when we come before Him in repentance.

In Isaiah 61, God promises His people beauty for ashes. As you release your stored grief, shame, guilt, and any emotions entwined; you may wish to personalize the following:

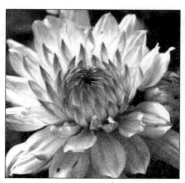

To appoint unto them that mourn in Zion, to give unto them beauty for ashes, the oil of joy for mourning, the garment of praise for the spirit of heaviness; that they might be called trees of righteousness, the planting of the LORD, that he might be glorified (Isa 61:3).

The Healthy Expression of Sorrow

This may consist of mourning for a period in whatever manner we need and accepting comfort from God and others with the expectation to heal and move forward after a time. We express gratefulness for what we had for a season and for the many blessings we still enjoy. We forgive where needed and release any guilt or shame involved so that we can move forward. God understands sorrow and grief. He gives us permission to cry and grieve for a time:

To everything there is a season, a time for every purpose under heaven: a time to weep, and a time to laugh; a time to mourn, and a time to dance (Eccl 3:1,4).

We all mourn and process loss in different ways. The following is an example of King David dealing with personal sorrow after the illness and death of his child. In this account, God previously made it plain that the child's illness was a direct result of David's sin of adultery and murder. David had prayed, fasted, and spent the night lying on the ground in search of God's mercy. However, after seven days the child died. Following his death:

> *David arose from the ground, washed and anointed himself, and changed his clothes; and he went into the house of the LORD and worshiped. Then he went to his own house; and when he requested, they set food before him, and he ate. Then his servants said to him, "What is this that you have done? You fasted and wept for the child while he was alive, but when the child died, you arose and ate food." And he said, "While the child was alive, I fasted and wept; for I said, 'Who can tell whether the LORD will be gracious to me, that the child may live?' But now he is dead; why should I fast? Can I bring him back again? I shall go to him, but he shall not return to me"*
> *(2 Sam 12:20-23).*

Many of us have experienced the impending death of a loved one. We may often mourn ahead of time as we come to terms with the idea of life without them. It is healthy to feel a sense of closure with the finality of death, and return to our routines.

In the Old Testament, the beloved Moses and his brother Aaron eventually died. The Israelite people freely mourned their deaths with tears for a set time before moving forward.

> *Now when all the congregation saw that Aaron was dead, all the house of Israel mourned for Aaron thirty days*
> *(Num 20-29).*

> *And the children of Israel wept for Moses in the plains of*

Moab thirty days. So the days of weeping and mourning for Moses ended (Deut 34:8).

Could prolonging sorrow in our lives only bring more suffering?
God's Word gives strength, hope, joy, and healing amid the heaviness of grief.

My soul melts from heaviness; strengthen me according to Your word (Ps 119:28).

And the ransomed of the LORD shall return, and come to Zion with singing, with everlasting joy on their heads. They shall obtain joy and gladness, and sorrow and sighing shall flee away (Isa 35:10).

God comforts His people who are mourning the physical death of a loved one. When death is put into proper perspective alongside life everlasting, we realize death is really a very short time of absence before a grand reunion.

But I do not want you to be ignorant, brethren, concerning those who have fallen asleep, lest you sorrow as others who have no hope. For if we believe that Jesus died and rose again, even so God will bring with Him those who sleep in Jesus. For this we say to you by the word of the Lord, that we who are alive and remain until the coming of the Lord will by 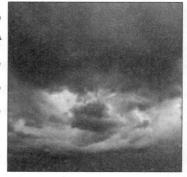 *no means precede those who are asleep. For the Lord*

Himself will descend from heaven with a shout, with the voice of an archangel, and with the trumpet of God. And the dead in Christ will rise first. Then we who are alive and remain shall be caught up together with them in the clouds to meet the Lord in the air. And thus we shall always be with the Lord. Therefore comfort one another with these words (I Thess 4:13-18).

If you are up there in age and Jesus is your Lord, do not think of yourself as closer to death. Rather think of yourself as that much closer to being made truly and fully alive!

At death, the Bible teaches that God's people are clothed in glorious immortality. Hope in this promise! Praise God for His gifts, even if some depart sooner than we would wish. Expressing joy and gratefulness aloud, though difficult at first, heals our hearts.

"And they shall come and shout for joy on the height of Zion, and they shall be radiant over the bounty of the LORD—over the grain, and the new wine, and the oil, and over the young of the flock and the herd; and their life shall be like a watered garden, and they shall never languish again (Jer 31:12, NASB®).

Note: The word languish is also translated sorrow.

There may be times when God allows us to experience grief when we fall out of step with Him. He reserves this right as a last resort, in loving hope that we might obediently return to Him.

Her adversaries have become her masters, her enemies prosper; for the LORD has caused her grief because of the multitude of her transgressions [...] (Lam 1:5, NASB®).

Now I rejoice, not that you were made sorry, but that your sorrow led to repentance. For you were made sorry in a godly manner, that you might suffer loss from us in nothing. For godly sorrow produces repentance leading to salvation, not to be regretted; but the sorrow of the world produces death (2 Cor 7:9-10).

When we see someone grieving over their life choices and seeking healthy change, we are called to go to them with compassion and love:

...on the contrary, you ought rather to forgive and comfort him, lest perhaps such a one be swallowed up with too much sorrow. Therefore I urge you to reaffirm your love to him (2 Cor 2: 7-8).

Sorrow, grief, and heartbreak are an inevitable part of this life. Please allow these emotions to fully process and release. Symbolic gestures and acts as well as allowing yourself to cry are all acceptable to God. We may need to mourn with others and receive their comfort and prayers. Replace the sorrows as they release with the good memories, lessons, joy, and gratefulness.

God does not want us to exhaust ourselves with prolonged grief and fall into depression and its accompanying physical ailments. Therefore, it is important to set a time to end our mourning and embrace the antidotes of joy, praise, and gratefulness. Together these restore health and energy to the whole body. Something I have observed is that those who have dealt with sorrows often seem to have greater capacity for mercy and compassion toward others going through difficult times.

Do you struggle finding joy in life? Joy is a journey. It is not based on everyday events like happiness is, but on living in the zone, that is, in the heart of the Father and in healthy alignment of mind, speech, emotions, lifestyle, service, truth, love, and intimacy with Him.

And these things we write to you that your joy may be full (I John 1:4, concerning all the Words of Life given by Jesus and recorded by the Apostles).

CONCLUSION CHECKLIST

____I commit to keeping my heart open to others and to God.

____I will set a time for mourning, during which I will freely express my sorrow and heartbreak.

____I will create rituals, memorials, or symbolic acts as needed to help sorrow release more easily.

____Though it may be difficult, I will consider spending time in thanksgiving, even during the first days of sorrow, and see how quickly this powerful grief neutralizer aids my healing.

____Everything I have is a gift, even my loved ones. I will express gratefulness to God for the days, weeks, or years I was given with them.

____I have told my loved ones what they mean to me so that I will have no regrets. I will consider writing a love letter to my parents, children, grandchildren, and other loved ones. (You may wish to frame this and give it as a gift.)

____I verbally express joy and gratefulness for what I have. I refuse to prolong sorrow and mourning by focusing on lost memories and milestones that I could have experienced. Instead, I claim God's beautiful gifts to replace all broken dreams and ashes in my life. I am determined to move forward.

____I will comfort others who are moving from sin and sorrow into a healthy relationship with God.

NOTES: _____

_____

_____

_____

_____

_____

_____

_____

_____

_____

_____

_____

_____

_____

_____

_____

_____

_____

_____

_____

_____

_____

_____

_____

_____

_____

_____

_____

_____

_____

VERBAL FREEDOM PRAYER FROM SORROW

I have decided to move on and release all mountains in my life.

In Jesus' name, by the authority of His Word, I command all mountains of sorrow, heartbreak, pain, depression, and grief, as well as any traumas, stories, or spiritual oppression to which these are connected, to be completely released from my entire being—especially from all physical parts that are depressed, cold, and sluggish. I command them from my life, birth, gestation, any connections to ancestors, genetics, thinking patterns, energies, emotional mechanisms, soul, and spirit.

I release grief from all molecules of my head, brain, neck, chest, central zone, pelvic zone, legs, immunity, bones and bone marrow, and all spinal parts.

I especially command these sorrows from energetic and cellular programming of my heart, its valves and heartbeat mechanisms, nerves, all veins and arteries, lymph, fat, blood pressure, lungs, bronchi, breathing mechanisms, diaphragm, eyes, and visual parts.

I am done with them! "Go to the feet of Jesus!" I forgive all men, women, children, myself, society, and God for any blame I carry regarding these emotions. The Son has set me free. I am free indeed! I claim this!

In the vacancies these create, I claim healthy physical,

emotional, mental, and spiritual patterns as God intended. I accept God's beauty and joy to take the place of death, loss, and any broken dreams in my life. I also fully receive into my whole being love, peace, patience, kindness, goodness, faithfulness, gentleness, self-control, forgiveness, gratefulness, God's comfort, and His good plans for me.

Thank you, Lord, for your healing provisions. Amen.

Important: read this slowly with intent and meaning. I have a framed anatomy chart to look at that I cut and pasted from an anatomy manual from a community college nearby. I highly recommend this to add sharpened focus and intention for serious challenges.

HEALING PEARL:
GOD'S SOLUTIONS TO FEAR, WORRY, AND ANXIETY

The Bible addresses fear in its various forms. Some fears are healthy and necessary while others hurt our health. In all forms, they are strong spurs for action.

One definition of fear is to have a healthy respect or awe towards something. Many times this is so that we may know our place and not overstep our boundaries. I have a healthy respect for the ocean, electricity, fire, and many other wonders of this earth. The Bible exhorts us many times to fear the Lord. This means we recognize God as mighty, powerful, and worthy of praise and obedience.

Unhealthy fear gives birth to paralyzing dread, worry, anxiety, tension, and stress. This may be a fear of failure, fear of success, fear of divorce, fear of marriage, fear of old age, fear of poverty, fear of illness, etc. Such fear usually partners with adrenaline excess (high stress response) that comes from waiting for that "lion" around the corner that often never materializes.

Fear of man is fear of how others may perceive and judge us. We are not to fear what others may think, especially when it pertains to our saying and doing the right thing. Neither unhealthy fear nor fear of man comes from God.

The fear of man brings a snare, but whoever trusts in the LORD shall be safe (Prov 29:25).

Listen to Me, you who know righteousness, you people in whose heart is My law: Do not fear the reproach of men, nor be afraid of their insults (Isa 51:7).

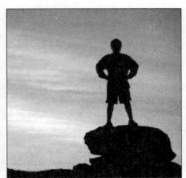

For He Himself has said, "I will never leave you nor forsake you." So we may boldly say: "The LORD is my helper; I will not fear. What can man do to me?" (Heb 13:5-6).

Fear affects us physically. Consider the interesting expressions we have coined: "yellow-bellied," "weak-kneed," and "spineless." We intuitively know that fear has a weakening effect on the kidneys: "He was so scared, he wet his pants."

In this study, we will associate fear and its companions mainly with muscle tension, the digestive organs, allergies (improper immune response), the kidneys and legs, as well as the heart and circulation.

The following Scriptures indicate that those who live in fear also live in a state of torment. When we do not reside in God's love, we give ground to unhealthy fears. When we fully accept God's gifts of power, love, and soundness of mind and fully trust in His remedies, even to the point of death and beyond, fear loses its power over us.

For God has not given us a spirit of fear, but of power and of love and of a sound mind (2 Tim 1:7).

There is no fear in love; but perfect love casts out fear, because fear involves torment. But he who fears has not been made perfect in love. We love Him because He first loved us (I Jn 4: 18-19).

Excessive Venting

If fear is something other than healthy respect or the quick response of self-protection, it can branch into unhealthy states of worry, anxiety, stress, and tension. Panic, indecisiveness, and rash decision-making may also manifest. Fear may even evolve into compulsive and overwhelming impulses, such as a strong and obsessive desire to lean on others excessively for advice and comfort. Some may be totally unaware of how exhausting their chronic venting patterns truly are to others.

The stomach reacts heavily to fear-based emotions. Digestion slows or stops as blood rushes to the extremities for action. We have all felt "butterflies" in our stomach, which sometimes may cause stomachaches. This is why we are told not to "worry ourselves into an ulcer." As adrenaline surges, it affects the nervous system. The throat, arteries, and muscles become tense and blood pressure rises. Under sudden, intense fear, muscles tremble, and the kidneys, spine, sciatic nerves, legs, knees, and ankles may suddenly weaken or become painful. The heart may even fail.

And the guards shook for fear of him, and became like dead men (Matt 28:4).

And so terrifying was the sight that Moses said, "I am exceedingly afraid and trembling" (Heb 12:21).

Men's hearts failing them from fear and the expectation of those things which are coming on the earth [...]
(Luke 21:26).

The substance cortisol, originating in the adrenals, rises from stress and is associated with excess belly fat, hormonal upsets, and suppressed immunity if unchecked over time. Chronic high cortisol can sabotage the body's ability to kill cancer cells.

Excessive tension and hyperactivity of hormones and organs may cycle with fatigue and exhaustion. Prostate issues, blood sugar imbalances, spastic colon, and water retention may commonly entwine with these.

The futility of worry and anxiety as well as their antidotes are made plain in God's Word:

> And which of you by worrying can add one cubit to his stature? If you then are not able to do the least, why are you anxious for the rest? Consider the lilies, how they grow: they neither toil nor spin; and yet I say to you, even Solomon in all his glory was not arrayed like one of these. If then God so clothes the grass, which today is in the field and tomorrow is thrown into the oven, 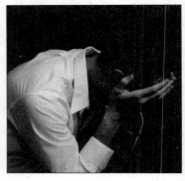 how much more will He clothe you, O you of little faith? And do not seek what you should eat or what you should drink, nor have an anxious mind. For all these things the nations of the world seek after, and your Father knows that you need these things. But seek the kingdom of God, and all these things shall be added to you (Luke 12:25-31).

Do you see the condition in the last verse above?

> Therefore humble yourselves under the mighty hand of God, that He may exalt you in due time, casting all your

care upon Him, for He cares for you (I Peter 5:6-7).

Please refer again to the Trauma Prayer in Appendix IV. Consider it as a powerful tool to release all types of fear strongholds, especially those relating to accidents, pain, injuries, birth trauma, shock, and terror of all types.

Suppressed Fear

Suppressed fear may come from not taking action, verbal or otherwise, against fear, worry, and anxiety, and instead stuffing them inside where a chronic physical pattern can result. Physical symptoms of suppressed fear may include skeletal and urinary imbalances, leg weakness, sexual weaknesses, headaches, fibromyalgia, various allergies, ulcers, excess belly fat, and various types of brain, nerve, adrenal, and spinal issues.

When Adam and Eve disobeyed God, they ran away and hid in fear. They could not bear to face God and their transparency and honesty were affected. Unhealthy communication is a common symptom of suppressed fear that can deteriorate even the best of relationships. When issues are left unresolved, they may give rise to guilt and shame.

Other manifestations may be withdrawal from community and an inability to accept love and intimacy from others and God. This is a downward spiral that may give way to addictions and a search for self-healing and comfort in all the wrong places: caffeine, nicotine, sugar, alcohol, overeating, prescription drugs, television, video games, pornography, etc.

Pastor Henry Wright who studies the spiritual roots of disease teaches that addiction is usually rooted in feeling a lack of love.[23] The first step to freedom is understanding the true love of God.

Habits are similar to addictions in that they are thoughts or actions that are repeatedly engaged. However, there is a key difference. One stops habits when learning they are wrong or harmful. On the other hand, one continues addictions, even after learning they are against God's plan and harmful to health.

God's antidotes that break addictions include building faith and intimacy with Him upon hearing His Word and fully accepting the perfect love He has to give us. Entwining these with personal integrity helps us into a state of freedom and wholeness that is more appealing than denial. One of my favorite affirmations is "I can do all things through Christ who strengthens me!" Here is a way to make use of this Scripture:

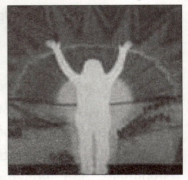

(Drawing Courtesy of Catherine Drauch Rogers)

"The Son has set me free. I am free indeed! I claim freedom from_____."

We can activate these Scriptures more fully by claiming them aloud several times daily until they have broken all strongholds. Resist Satan and harness the power of God's Words!

Healthy Expression of Fear

The healthy expression of fear involves both a feeling and an action. First it is a healthy respect for what is powerful, both in this world and in the heavens. This then becomes a springboard for wise action toward these things.

The fear of the LORD is the beginning of wisdom [...] (Prov 9:10).

When we develop a sense of healthy respect for God and His authority over creation, we are more inclined to obey Him. Fear of the Lord turns us from evil, physically strengthens us, and yields tremendous blessings.

> But the mercy of the LORD is from everlasting to everlasting on those who fear Him, and His righteousness to children's children, to such as keep His covenant, and to those who remember His commandments to do them (Ps 103:17-18).

> The fear of the LORD prolongs days [...] (Prov 10:27).

> [...] And by the fear of the LORD one departs from evil. When a man's ways please the LORD, He makes even his enemies to be at peace with him (Prov 16:6-7).

Three Stages of Spiritual Growth

I was taught this insightful tool in college. Where do you feel you reside?

Stage 1: Fear of Punishment This involves coming into obedience to God out of healthy respect and awe of His power to create, destroy, and pass righteous judgment.

Stage 2: Desire for Reward This involves following God's will for our lives as we recognize the joy-filled rewards of doing so.

Stage 3: Honoring God This involves full maturity. We stay in His will not because of what he can do for us, but because we love and honor Him for who He is as our loving Creator.

As children, we moved through similar stages with our parents if we have healthy relationships with them.

God's Willingness to be Our Shield and Protector

God promises to protect and comfort those who follow Him in faith so that they may know His peace.

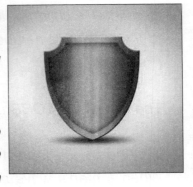

After these things the word of the LORD came to Abram in a vision, saying, "Do not be afraid, Abram. I am your shield [...] (Gen 15:1).

And Moses said to the people, "Do not be afraid. Stand still, and see the salvation of the LORD, which He will accomplish for you today. For the Egyptians whom you see today, you shall see again no more forever. The LORD will fight for you, and you shall hold your peace" (Ex 14:13-14).

And when the servant of the man of God arose early and went out, there was an army, surrounding the city with horses and chariots. And his servant said to him, "Alas, my master! What shall we do?" So he answered, "Do not fear, for those who are with us are more than those who are with them." And Elisha prayed, and said, "LORD, I pray, open his eyes that he may see." Then the LORD opened the eyes of the young man, and he saw. And behold, the mountain was full of horses and chariots of fire all around Elisha (2 Kings 6:15-17).

And I commanded Joshua at that time, saying, "Your eyes have seen all that the LORD your God has done to these two kings; so will the LORD do to all the kingdoms through which you pass. You must not fear them, for the LORD your God Himself fights for you" (Deut 3:21:22).

As a Christian, claim God as your shield and protector. In faith, claim His protection over your life, home, car, and job. Do not give in to fear and its insecurity else you lose sight of God's promise to care for you. If you are harboring doubt in your life, what is creating it? Give it to the Lord. God promises to carry us one hundred percent of every minute of every day. Believe it. Reach out and receive it.

If you are searching for peace in God, reaffirm the following aloud:

For I am persuaded that neither death nor life, nor angels nor principalities nor powers, nor things present nor things to come, nor height nor depth, nor any other created thing, shall be able to separate us from the love of God which is in Christ Jesus our Lord (Rom 8:38-39).

These things I have spoken to you, that in Me you may have peace. In the world you will have tribulation; but be of good cheer, I have overcome the world" (John 16:33).

The decision to place our trust in God as our shield and protector dispels fear. Even in times of tragedy or death, we can take courage because God promises to work for the good of those who love Him.

The LORD will not allow the righteous to hunger, but He will thrust aside the craving of the wicked (Prov 10:3).

I would have lost heart, unless I had believed that I would see the goodness of the LORD in the land of the living. Wait on the LORD; be of good courage, and He shall strengthen your heart; wait, I say, on the LORD (Ps 27:13-14)!

Yea, though I walk through the valley of the shadow of death, I will fear no evil; for You are with me; Your rod and Your staff, they comfort me (Ps 23:4)!

Strengthen the weak hands, and make firm the feeble knees. Say to those who are fearful-hearted, "Be strong, do not fear (Isa 35:3-4)!

The steps of a man are established by the LORD; and He delights in his way. When he falls, he shall not be hurled headlong; because the LORD is the One who holds his hand (Ps 37:23-24, NASB®).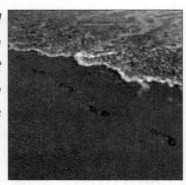

Once we come to grips with our fears by claiming God's promises, taking courage, and realizing that He is willing to love and walk beside us, we truly break the worst fear of all—that of physical death. For the faithless, death can be the worst truth about life; for the believer, it is a glorious upgrade.

Share all of your experiences with God so that He becomes your partner in solving life's challenges. Take what actions you feel you can handle and transfer the remaining burden to our Heavenly Father's willing shoulders. Walk in courage and confidence, safe and secure in His unfailing love.

HEALING PEARL:
THE VALUE OF CONTENTMENT

Managing fears properly and trusting God's strength and provision lead to contentment.

> *Now godliness with contentment is great gain. For we brought nothing into this world, and it is certain we can carry nothing out. And having food and clothing, with these we shall be content (I Tim 6:6-8).*

> *[...] I have learned in whatever state I am, to be content: I can do all things through Christ who strengthens me (Phil 4:11,13).*

> *Let your character be free from the love of money, being content with what you have; for He Himself has said, "I will never desert you, nor will I ever forsake you," so that we confidently say, "The Lord is my helper, I will not be afraid. What shall man do to me?" (Heb 13:5-6, NASB®).*

Diligently pursue emotional health, putting the various verbal exercises mentioned in this chapter to the test. Watch as your body relaxes and heals as old layers of unresolved emotions and torment clear and free you to conform to God's intended healthy patterns.

I have never witnessed a tool more powerful than processing these truths weekly in a group of like-minded people, together proclaiming emotional freedom from any areas of concern; and praying and claiming God's principles from His Word.

Tough Patterns

I have found that a tough pattern releases best when I label the issue a "mountain" and command it to leave "the energetic and cellular programming of my brain and entire being" (as well as naming any other desired body parts using anatomy pictures) and "my life, birth, all genetics, and any iniquities passed from my entire lineage back to the beginning of time." These quoted phrases are very important and worth adding to any prayer of release that you compose. The phrases can already be found in the Freedom Prayers in this chapter. Consider praying these regularly until peace returns.

I have made a comforting observation that long-standing health issues that have taken a long time to build into serious challenges may sometimes release relatively quickly with this work. Henry Wright has written of the same observation.

Maintenance

When you are consistently feeling well, consider more abbreviated releases. I do them first thing in the morning if I do not feel at peace. I replace what I release with healthy affirmations, Scriptures, and "God's patterns for total, perfect health."

CONCLUSION CHECKLIST

____I can explain the difference between healthy and unhealthy fear.

____I will aim to please God first and foremost by confronting, head-on, my fear of what others may think. My God is my refuge. What can man truly do to me?

____I remind myself when needed, "It is none of my business what others think of me."

____I am committed to changing worry and anxiety into healthy choices and actions. I cannot predict the future. I prepare for it, but I release all fear and worry into God's hands as I claim His promises of care for me. If I have been trying to be Controller of the Universe, I am considering today my retirement.

____I have prayerfully and verbally dedicated my health, children, home, car, and business to God as the true owner. He knows how to take better care of His property than I do. I still do my reasonable part, but for the rest, I take refuge in Him. I learn to trust in God's perfect timing.

____In my workplace, I am God's employee and work at my best to please Him. I promote my business reasonably. I put the ultimate success or failure of my business into God's hands.

____I am determined to take courage, verbally if needed, to make the best decisions that bring the greatest sense of integrity and peace.

____I remind myself to live in the present moment to combat any worry or anxiety of the future.

____I assess my maturity level with God. Is my relationship currently founded upon a healthy respect for God's power, justice, and a love for who He is (His nature and attributes), or simply on the anticipation of reward and fear of punishment?

____I visualize God holding my hand daily until we meet face to face.

Homework: Copy and laminate the three Freedom Prayers, Appendix III, and the Trauma Prayer in Appendix IV. Consider speaking them every one to two weeks. Spend some quiet time and honestly evaluate where you are in your journey. Ask God to give you insight and wisdom in what more needs to be done and verbally address them.

NOTES: _____

VERBAL FREEDOM PRAYER FROM FEAR AND ANXIETY

I am determined to move forward by releasing all mountains in my life.

In Jesus' name and upon the authority of His Word, I command all mountains of shock, trauma, injury, anxiety, addiction, worry, fear, and malfunctions of any types, as well as all forms of spiritual oppression, to come out of wherever they have attached to my being—all molecules of my head, brain, neck, chest, central zone, pelvic zone, legs, nerves, immunity, bones, and bone marrow—and be sent to the feet of Jesus. I am done with them!

I especially address all energetic and cellular programming of my heart, digestive organs, kidneys, bladder, urethra, adrenal glands, spine, disks, neck and spinal cord, lymph, blood vessels, unwanted fat, muscles, cartilage, tendons and ligaments, and especially all parts of my knees, ankles and legs, as well as all tense, constricted, or hyperactive areas.

I command them from my mind and spirit, as well as from my entire life, birth, gestation, and any imprinting from any source, including all genetics and iniquities from my mother's and father's lineages back to all generations.

I ask forgiveness for holding fear and its offspring, and I forgive all whom I may blame.

In their vacancies, I claim healthy physical, mental,

emotional, and spiritual patterns as God intended for me, and a healing miracle if needed.

I fully accept God's courage, power, protection, comfort, love, joy, peace, patience, kindness, faithfulness, self-control, and a sound mind to flood my entire being. The Son has set me free, I am free indeed!

Thank you, Lord. Amen.

Consider speaking the above prayer two to four times monthly, or when needed, along with the Trauma Release Prayer in Appendix IV.

CLAIRE'S PRAYER

Father, God, I ask you to forgive and cleanse me for participating with that (fear, thought, worry, stress, anxiety, or tension) just now. I repent and renounce that thought and the spirit of fear.

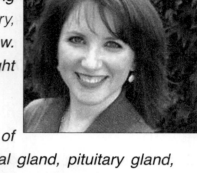

Spirit of fear, I break you off of my hypothalamus, thyroid, pineal gland, pituitary gland, nerves, central and parasympathetic nervous systems, cardiovascular system, every piece and part of my body, and out of all energetic and cellular programming of my body.

In the name of Jesus Christ of Nazareth (the Word of God in the flesh), I command fear to let loose of my mind, body, soul, and spirit and go where the Lord Jesus tells you to go and never return!

Body, I speak to my hypothalamus. I direct you to settle down, release all fear, and return to normal levels. Body, be in a state of peace right now. I direct all hormones, including cortisol and adrenaline, to go to normal levels right now in Jesus' name. Body, return to peace in Jesus. He has not given you a spirit of fear but of power, love, and sound mind.

Perfect love casts out fear and Jesus is perfect love. In Jesus' name. Amen.

Claire has an amazing testimony of healing regarding the nervous system of her throat, in which her throat would spasm and close when eating. She had tried many medical and natural approaches for years, but this prayer that she composed (before this book was written) began working immediately as she developed her prayer more completely for what she needed. She inspired many in my first class.

Part 4
Pearls of Spiritual Health

S PIRITUAL HEALTH is described in God's Word as the development of Christ-like qualities within our spirit. Faith, hope, love, and discernment of truth are examples of such qualities. As our spiritual self evolves, our selfish desires dissolve. Every decision we make influences our spiritual health.

Our spirit is made in the likeness of God's Spirit—with emotions, reason, and life force. Life has a way of refining and testing us to continually reflect where our level of maturity lies and how adept we have become in rightly handling God's Word for our challenges.

HEALING PEARL:
GOD WANTS US TO BE HIS MASTERPIECE

Those who pursue the spiritual heavenly realm as their eternal goal are committed to maturing in relationship with God and walking in His truth.

God, in His love for us, will refine and test us through the inevitable trials of life. These will work to our good when we keep our focus on love and obedience to Him.

> *I will [...] refine them as silver is refined, And test them as gold is tested. They will call on My name, and I will answer them. I will say, "This is My people'; and each one will say, 'The LORD is my God" (Zech 13:9).*

HEALING PEARL:
GOD HAS GIVEN US HIS PRECIOUS PROMISES

If we invite our Heavenly Father to have His way with us and we humbly and joyfully accept His conditions and promises, we will become the masterpieces He intended.

> *[...] As His divine power has given to us all things that pertain to life and godliness, through the knowledge of Him who called us by glory and virtue, by which have been given to us exceedingly great and precious promises [...] (2 Pet 1:3-4).*

HEALING PEARL:
HAVE FAITH IN WHAT GOD CAN DO

Hearing builds faith. I am convinced that God meant His Words to be read aloud as a treatment for our entire being. God's words also bring life and health to our flesh. Please make reading the Bible aloud a priority if you are not feeling well.

> *So then faith comes by hearing, and hearing by the word*

of God (Rom 10-17).

But without faith it is impossible to please Him, for he who comes to God must believe that He is, and that He is a rewarder of those who diligently seek Him (Heb 11:6).

It takes time sometimes to build faith. Is your faith suffering? Ask for more of it! This man was not faulted for his request:

Then one of the crowd answered and said, "Teacher, I brought You my son, who has a mute spirit. And wherever he seizes him, he throws him down; he foams at the mouth, gnashes his teeth, and becomes rigid. So I spoke to Your disciples, that they should cast him out, but they could not." He answered him and said, "O faithless generation, how long shall I be with you? How long shall I bear with you? Bring him to Me." Then they brought him to Him. And when he saw Him, immediately the spirit convulsed him, and he fell on the ground...So He asked his father, "How long has this been happening to him?" And he said, "From childhood. And often he has thrown him both into the fire and into the water to destroy him. But if You can do anything, have compassion on us and help us." Jesus said to him, "If you can believe, all things are possible to him who believes." Immediately the father of the child cried out and said with tears, "Lord, I believe; help my unbelief" (Mark 9:17-24)!

Faith, belief, and Jesus' name opens portals to the miraculous. Next, Jesus has some wisdom for His apostles regarding their lack of success:

So Jesus said to them, "Because of your unbelief; for assuredly, I say to you, if you have faith as a mustard seed, you will say to this mountain, 'Move from here to there,' and it will move; and nothing will be impossible for you. However, this kind does not go out except by prayer and fasting" (Matt 17:20-21).

It is interesting that this "mountain" needed prayer and fasting to assist its removal. Following are more Scriptures citing the necessity of belief:

And when He had come into the house, the blind men came to Him. And Jesus said to them, "Do you believe that I am able to do this?" They said to Him, "Yes, Lord." Then He touched their eyes, saying, "According to your faith let it be to you." And their eyes were opened (Matt 9:28-30).

But Jesus looked at them and said, "With men it is impossible, but not with God; for with God all things are possible" (Mark 10:27).

This is why we also feel free to ask God for a creative miracle if He chooses to give it.

And on the basis of faith in His name, it is the name of Jesus which has strengthened this man whom you see and know; and the faith which comes through Him has given him this perfect health in the presence of you all (Acts 3:16, NASB®).

Once you are committed to a course of faith in prayer and proclamation, carefully guard against thoughts, actions, or words that negate your faith. Do not practice or speak doubt and unbelief.

Two farmers prayed for rain. One immediately went out and prepared his fields. The other did not. Which farmer are you?[24]

HEALING PEARL:
GOD GIVES US HIS PROTECTION

Are you ready to face the giants in your life? As you lay down your baggage, take up your tools of offense. This life is meant to be one of victory.

Therefore take up the whole armor of God, that you may be able to withstand in the evil day, and having done all, to stand. Stand therefore, having girded your waist with truth, having put on the breastplate of righteousness, and having shod your feet with the preparation of the gospel of peace; above all, taking the shield of faith with which you will be able to quench all the fiery darts of the wicked one. And take the helmet of salvation, and the sword of the Spirit, which is the word of God (Eph 6:13-17).

No weapon formed against you shall prosper, And every tongue which rises against you in judgment You shall condemn. This is the heritage of the servants of the LORD, And their righteousness is from Me,"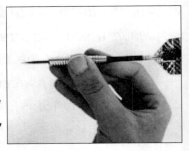

Says the LORD (Isa 54:17).

If you are a servant of the Lord, these are your power verses! Is your body being attacked with an illness? Consider boldly proclaiming daily, "No weapon including *(insert name of illness)* formed against me shall prosper!" Name the body parts to which you wish to apply this and the condition you want vanquished.

God's Promises to the Tither

Christians usually agree that tithing is giving a tenth of our income to the church for the Lord's service. Tithing supports the church, its staff, community outreach, and missions. Often, how we view money is a reflection of the hardness or softness of our hearts. In the verse below, the devourer may be anything that devours or threatens to rob our protection and peace in God: i.e. disasters, disease, theft, etc. It contains a conditional promise that might begin to explain why there is so much famine, suffering, and poverty in the world.

Bring all the tithes into the storehouse, that there may be food in My house, and try Me now in this," says the LORD of hosts, "if I will not open for you the windows of heaven and pour out for you such blessing that there will not be room enough to receive it. "And I will rebuke the devourer for your sakes, so that he will not destroy the fruit of your ground, nor shall the vine fail to bear fruit for you in the field," says the LORD of hosts; "and all nations will call you blessed, for you will be a delightful land," says the LORD of hosts (Mal 3:10-12).

Next we read of a promise to the charitable that may be a more protective health insurance policy than we currently own. When we take time (hopefully regularly) to give love, compassion, and mercy to those less fortunate, God notices.

> *How blessed is he who considers the helpless; the LORD will deliver him in a day of trouble.* 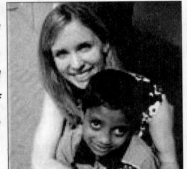 *The LORD will protect him, and keep him alive, and he shall be called blessed upon the earth; and do not give him over to the desire of his enemies. The LORD will sustain him upon his sickbed; in his illness, Thou dost restore him to health.*
> *--Ps 41:1-3 (NASB®)*

When you are serving others, claim this wonderful promise.

HEALING PEARL:
GOD GIVES US EVERY TOOL WE NEED

Paul claimed the following to give him strength when life was tough.

> *I can do all things through Christ who strengthens me* (Phil 4:13).

There is nothing we cannot endure or overcome with God's help. Confess to God your weaknesses. Proclaim His strength over them. Is there a weapon raised against you on any level? Stand up to it. Claim your adoption as God's child. Let your faith build by reading Scripture aloud. Choose, affirm, and claim His promises daily. Speak out the emotional baggage. Clean out personal cobwebs that clog your conscience. Ask others to pray with you and lay hands upon you. Thank God ahead of time for sending healing and victory your way!

HEALING PEARL:
GOD SHOWS US HOW TO BE AT OUR BEST

God has showered us with His wisdom on a multi-faceted approach to health. Wise men of old praise the life and health of His teachings.

> *O LORD, by these things men live; and in all these things is the life of my spirit; so You will restore me and let me live (Isa 38:16).*

> *For they are life to those who find them, And health to all their flesh (Prov 4:22).*

God also shows us how to avoid stumbling into psychic pain, injury, and trauma:

> *But also for this very reason, giving all diligence, add to your faith virtue, to virtue knowledge, to knowledge self-control, to self-control perseverance, to perseverance godliness, to godliness brotherly kindness, and to brotherly kindness love. For if these things are yours and abound, you will be neither barren nor unfruitful in the knowledge of our Lord Jesus Christ. For he who lacks these things is*

short-sighted, even to blindness, and has forgotten that he was cleansed from his old sins. Therefore, brethren, be even more diligent to make your call and election sure, for if you do these things you will never stumble [...] (2 Pet 1:5-10).

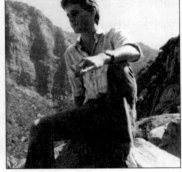

Beloved, I pray that you may prosper in all things and be in health, just as your soul prospers (3 John 2).

Our health and its prosperity appears strongly connected to our soul's health.

HEALING PEARL:
THE RECIPE FOR PEACE IN THIS LIFE

True peace is profound. It is independent of everyday life as we lose our ties to earthly things and embrace our spiritual journey of love and intimacy with our Heavenly Father. He desires for our spirit to be at peace regardless of life's ups and downs. He is constantly molding and refining us. He gives us instructions that are instrumental in bringing about our active participation and growth. These instructions make us relational and responsible.

Rejoice in the Lord always. Again I will say, rejoice! Let your gentleness be known to all men. The Lord is at hand. Be anxious for nothing, but in everything by prayer and supplication, with thanksgiving, let your requests be made known to God; and the peace of God, which surpasses all understanding, will guard your hearts and minds through Christ Jesus. Finally, brethren, whatever things are true, whatever things are noble, whatever things are just, whatever things are pure, whatever things are lovely, whatever things are of good report, if there is any virtue and if there is anything praiseworthy—meditate on these things. The things which you learned and received and heard and saw in me, these do, and the God of peace will be with you (Phil 4:4-9).

HEALING PEARL:
THE PRINCIPLE OF DAILY GRATEFULNESS

What would you give for a fountain of youth? There is actually a youth-renewing set of Bible verses. Could youthfulness be a by-product of gratefulness? The emotion of gratefulness has a miraculous impact upon the molecular structure of water and, we might also conclude, upon our own bodies, which are 80% water. To bless is to speak well of. Bless our glorious God daily. Bless others. Bless yourself. Personalize the Scripture below. Write down its benefits and claim them each day with gratitude:

Bless the LORD, O my soul; and all that is within me, bless His holy name! Bless the LORD, O my soul, and forget not all His benefits: Who forgives all your iniquities, Who heals all your diseases, Who redeems your life from destruction, Who crowns you with lovingkindness and tender mercies, Who satisfies your mouth with good things, so that your youth is renewed like the eagle's (Ps 103-1-5).

I love this verse. I have it posted where I can read it daily aloud. It restores my strength and peace when life is overwhelming.

The Middle and Golden Years

For those of you in your middle and golden years, you may wish to apply the following verse to your life. Notice there is speaking involved.

They shall still bear fruit in old age; They shall be fresh and flourishing, To declare that the LORD is upright; He is my rock, and there is no unrighteousness in Him (Ps 92:14-15).

Consider keeping these verses on your refrigerator or mirror to speak daily, remember how truly blessed you are, and remind yourself of the exciting life to which God has called you.

CONCLUSION CHECKLIST

____I have made the decision to accept nothing less than God's best for my life. This applies to the friends, dates, and mate that I choose.

____I will rid my life of 'tolerations' that distract from my goals-- *stuff* that clutters my time and energies at home or work. If I have not looked at or had any contact with my *stuff* within the last year, I will get rid of it. It is time to clean out my office, closets, garage, car, and home.

____I am becoming familiar with God's promises. I look to see if there are conditions that I must meet for them to be fulfilled.

____I am not ashamed to ask God to help me build my faith, understanding, and wisdom.

____I attend church as God requests and tithe out of obedience and gratitude. I claim God's promise that He will rebuke the devourer of my resources. If an issue of loss arises, I will first check my integrity then claim this promise and confront the issue. I will trust God for rectification in His timing.

____I am determining a way to cheerfully assist the helpless and poor each month, above my tithe, as an offering of love to the Lord. I will claim God's health promises that pertain to this.

____I am rejoicing as my youth is renewed by a life that conforms to God's will and goodness as I daily bless God and express my gratefulness.

____I will dwell on the good in life, others, and God. I demonstrate love to all.

____I will be on the offense against all evil raised against me. I will claim victory as I wisely use the tools God has given. I will verbally proclaim Scripture over myself, family, and home as a start. If I am conscious of any sin in my life, I will use God's tools to stop it.

____I understand that God created me with the ability to choose. Each day I say "yes" or "no" to many things. These choices shape my spiritual health and maturity.

____I am on guard against any enticement that leads me into sin and away from God's blessings. I commit to staying in the blessing zone. God's vision for my life is far better than my own.

____I am discerning between Satan's whisperings, my natural inclinations, God's prompting, and the healthier spiritual level of response when I evaluate all incoming thoughts and resulting decisions.

____I am nurturing and encouraging excellence in myself and others.

____I will surrender every stress to God as it arises. I will make Him my partner in life.

____I will share my pearls lovingly with those who need God's health in their lives. I willingly share my testimony as a powerful witness that can encourage others.

NOTES: _____

_____

_____

_____

_____

_____

_____

_____

_____

_____

_____

_____

_____

_____

_____

_____

_____

_____

_____

_____

_____

_____

_____

_____

_____

_____

_____

_____

_____

_____

_____

Part 5
Using Your Pearls

Now that you have collected your pearls, begin using them for victory in your life. Here is a quick review:

Be Conscious of Your Physical Habits

You are worthy of health! Eat whole foods. Drink clean water. Exercise and rest properly. Make friends and have a social identity. Find a passion in your life. These all contribute positively to health.

Regularly pray aloud over your food and water as well as all vaccines, dental materials, and medications. In Jesus' name, command all negative components that they may contain to neutralize and become harmless to your body. Express daily gratefulness to God for your food, shelter, and clothing.

Please be aware that continuing health-destroying habits like smoking, recreational drugs, or excessive alcohol consumption, while asking God for healing of the diseases they produce can be futile. These are like inviting Death into one's life in small daily doses. I believe God allows our choices and the consequences they bring, which may unfortunately block God's life-giving blessings.

Do not be overcome by evil, but overcome evil with good (Rom 12:21).

Because of the above verse, I have made a commitment to use health-promoting remedies within my knowledge base in overcoming imbalances and disease in my life when at all possible. I believe a loving God has made provision in this area. I also believe He opens new doors of opportunity if I need to expand my options. It is always prudent to evaluate every remedy for its potential, both for harm and for good.

Be Conscious of Your Thoughts

Read God's Word daily, preferably in the morning so as to provide a great foundation for the day. Take all thoughts captive and do not accept them without evaluation. What you adopt and think, you will become. Hold high expectations for your life.

Utilize Bible verses and principles to free yourself from any imprinted or inherited mental patterns that do not promote health. When you speak aloud and incorporate new truths, you stimulate new information, holding neurons to form in the brain. Live in the present. Cultivate a joy for the future.

Be Conscious of Your Emotions

Determine to rid yourself of all past emotional baggage, plus all traumas (which have elements of shock, terror, injury, and pain) from your present, past, birth, gestation, and any inherited genetics and iniquities. This can take time. You did not get to where you are overnight. It takes time to peel off the 'onion layers.'

Daily, take a few minutes to meditate on anything that is interfering with your peace that day, and take action. Unresolved emotions resolve when appropriate action is taken. Speaking aloud is also an action. As you release old patterns, always replace them with healthy ones.

Pray over your children and your pets. If a living being cannot pray out loud or comprehend how to do this, you can pray aloud over them. It works!

Enlist others to help you if you have a particularly resistant pattern or strong sinful inclinations.

Satan may very well be a legalist. From repeated evidence in biofeedback, it appears that he may not release his hold on you until you name the enslavement and command it out.

You can learn to fight him more effectively by naming the specific issues binding you as well as the specific body parts affected. Use an anatomy book to help you. If we have not guarded ourselves with God's Word against him, he may have breached unguarded areas in our lives and have a sort of legal right to enslave us in various areas, including our health. (If you have a lack of knowledge here, ask the Lord for wisdom.) I often spend time naming issues, body parts, several emotions, and trauma to clear an issue and regain what I have lost. There is power in naming names!

A group gathered together for restoration, healing, and prayer is very powerful. Affirm Jesus as your helper. Remember what He said when we gather as a group in His name:

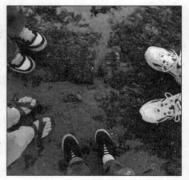

For where two or three are gathered together in my name, I am there in the midst of them (Matt 18-20).

Praying over each other with Christ in attendance is powerful! In my classes, we command out the mountains that we want removed and claim God's perfect patterns in its place. If we pray and proclaim according to God's will, He promises to hear us. It is easier to pray according to His will when we become proficient in the study of His Word.

If something comes to mind that we feel we should pray about, we do it. We also ask for God's wisdom in what to pray against. We listen for what each individual wants to address and pray it over or out of their life, gestation and birth, and genetics. We take key Scriptures and affirm them daily for continued healing.

I have seen many amazing health shifts occur in just two to four weeks when daily using Scriptures and affirmations.

Be confident that your faith will build over time by putting the principles in this book to the test. Grab hold of all your pearls and weave them throughout your life's tapestry.

Learn to Create and Compose Your Own Simple Prayers When You Need Them Quickly

Lynn, who inspired my class with her insightful writings and prayers, was happy to contribute a helpful tool she composed. She releases emotions in prayer as she thinks the word SAFE.

S = Sorrow
A = Anger
F = Fear
E = Emotions of Unforgiveness

She then fills the space left behind with healthy patterns. Remember that life and death is in the power of the tongue.

The SAFE acronym allows one to pray quickly when in

difficult situations while experiencing calmness through God's Holy Spirit.

Class Question

In one class, I was asked how one would deal with insomnia from a Biblical perspective. I used a Bible concordance to search the Scriptures using the key word "sleep." I noted that the Scriptures contains many clues as to what contributes to proper sleep and what deters from it. See the results in Appendix V. One can find many Godly answers to life's challenges by using this format and literally praying the elements of Scripture over any weakness as well as taking appropriate action.

Anticipate Satan's attack, especially in your thought life, and his accusing words. Remember his mission is to kill, steal, and destroy. Several of us had tough health issues and life challenges that appeared suddenly, challenging our newfound pearls. Satan does not like the application of this material. Persevere anyway! The stronger you become in God's Word, the better your spiritual immunity against him.

Stay faithful and work patiently as you witness God's gifts of beauty for ashes taking place.

Do not be timid. I rarely prayed aloud before this study, and then all at once I had to do so as the leader. It did not take long to release my fear as I relaxed and took refuge in the confidence that God wanted me to grow in this manner.

God is not ashamed to be called our God, even with all the mistakes we have made in our lives. We should not be timid then to proclaim Him or His truth. He is mighty and Holy and full of love for us, and He invites us to spend eternity with Him! He is worthy of all our devotion.

Introduce this material to your church, Bible study, retreat group or simply invite your friends and neighbors. We have work to do and a world to change. God bless you and be with you always!

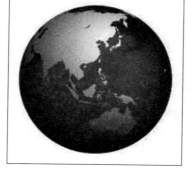

NOTES: _____

_____

_____

_____

_____

_____

_____

_____

_____

_____

_____

_____

_____

_____

_____

_____

_____

_____

_____

_____

_____

_____

_____

_____

_____

_____

_____

_____

_____

_____

_____

_____

Appendix I

The Salvation Blueprint

For by grace you have been saved through faith, and that not of yourselves; it is the gift of God, not of works, lest anyone should boast. For we are His workmanship [...] (Eph 2:8-10).

And it shall come to pass that whoever calls on the name of the LORD shall be saved (Acts 2:21).

Calling on the name of the Lord is acknowledging Him as our Maker, Savior, and Judge. It is an appeal to His mercy, love, and compassion. Here we reach upward to God.

The Apostle Peter explains the full process of salvation when talking to devout Jews. He defines what they must do to become Christians (Christ followers). It is no different for us. Because we are not saved by our own works, none of Peter's instructions are a work of humanity. Salvation is a work of God.

Men of Israel, hear these words: Jesus of Nazareth, a Man attested by God to you by miracles, wonders, and signs which God did through Him in your midst, as you yourselves also know—Him, being delivered by the determined purpose and foreknowledge of God, you have taken by lawless hands, have crucified, and put to death; whom God raised up, having loosed the pains of death, because it was not possible that He should be held by it [...] this Jesus, God has raised up, of which we are all witnesses. Therefore being exalted to the right hand of God, and having received from the Father the promise of the Holy Spirit, He poured out this which you now see and hear [...] Therefore let all the house of Israel know assuredly that God has made this Jesus, whom you crucified, both Lord and Christ (Acts 2:22-24, 32-33, 36)

Notice the hearers' response of convicting, active belief—belief that demanded action.

Now when they heard this, they were cut to the heart, and said to Peter and the rest of the apostles, "Men and brethren, what shall we do?" (Acts 2:37).

Peter did not yet confirm that they were saved or that their sins were forgiven. True belief results in action. The Scriptures teach we must obey the Good News (the Gospel) to be saved.

Then Peter said to them, "Repent, and let every one of you be baptized in the name of Jesus Christ for the remission of sins; and you shall receive the gift of the Holy Spirit. For the promise is to you and to your children, and to all who are afar off, as many as the Lord our God will call"
(Acts 2:37-39).

The remission of sins means the forgiveness of sins resulting in a clear conscience before God.

Forgiveness of sins is linked above to repentance and baptism. In all cases of conversion after Christ's death, baptism is taught to follow immediately so as to not delay this important step.

Then those who gladly received his word were baptized; and that day about three thousand souls were added to them (Acts 2:41).

And now why are you waiting? Arise and be baptized, and wash away your sins, calling on the name of the Lord (Acts 22:16).

Salvation results from active belief in Jesus and from obeying the Gospel. Salvation is both a moment in one's life and a process that God completes at the end of time as we remain vigilant in our obedience to Him.

When the Lord Jesus is revealed from heaven with His mighty angels, in flaming fire taking vengeance on those who do not know God, and on those who do not obey the gospel of our Lord Jesus Christ (2 Thess 1:7-9).

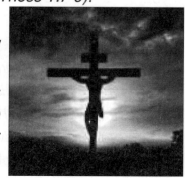

We are to re-enact symbolically Christ's death, burial and resurrection, signifying our death to our self-governed life and our entrance into newness of life in Christ. In other words, we do symbolically what He did in reality.

We repent, die to our old life of sin, and bury it in baptism, where our sins are washed away, and we rise to a new life, clothed with Christ. God sees us as His adopted children, joint-heirs of eternal life with His Son, Jesus.

> For you are all sons of God through faith in Christ Jesus. For as many of you as were baptized into Christ have put on Christ (Gal 3:26-27).

We rise out of the water to live a new life of transformation that is pleasing to God.

There is only one Gospel or Good News presented after the death of Christ by which we are called Christians. After Christ's resurrection, every person in God's Word who accepted the salvation message had obeyed the Gospel. It is important to understand the path to salvation. Always measure man's teaching against the Scriptures.

> But even if we, or an angel from heaven, preach any other gospel to you than what we have preached to you, let him be accursed (Gal 1:8).

If your heart is ready, reach up to the Lord in prayer. He is ready to welcome you home.

> Dear Heavenly Father,
> By faith on your promises, I choose to enter into salvation covenant with You. I believe Jesus is the Christ, Your Son, sent to offer salvation to mankind. I confess I have sinned. I am ready to repent of my old lifestyle and self-

governed thinking and accept Your instruction, capable of transforming my entire being. I am ready to be immersed with Christ in Christian baptism, taking part symbolically in the likeness of His death, that I may likewise take part in the coming resurrection. I pray sincerely and gratefully in Your Son's Holy name.

Amen.

Seek out a Christian Church. Tell them of your prayer, decision, and desire to be baptized. You will be joining a great body of believers whom God is daily transforming into the masterpieces He intended.

Appendix II

Tools for Cleansing

What follows are common emotional groups that, when unresolved, may be strong factors in holding us in bondage to disease. The words typed in capitol letters are the most common ones addressed, but they may be of no less importance.

FEAR	lust
WORRY	shyness
ANXIETY	insecurity
TERROR	meddling, bossiness
STRESS/TENSION	lying
FRIGHT	greed
SHOCK	envy
TRAUMA	covetousness
ACCIDENT TRAUMA	paralysis in moving forward

UNFORGIVENESS OF SELF, WOMEN, MEN, CHILDREN, SOCIETY, OR GOD	BITTERNESS RESENTMENT BLAME

SORROW	despair
GRIEF	hopelessness
HEARTBREAK	excessive vulnerability
PAIN	possessiveness
SHAME	neediness
GUILT	self-pity
DEPRESSION	selfishness
LONELINESS	withdrawal from others
ABANDONMENT	dependency
REJECTION	

ANGER	critical spirit
RAGE	slander
EXTREME HATRED	gossip
BETRAYAL	rejection
impatience	condemnation
rebelliousness	revenge
desire to control others	violence
jealousy	cursing others/oneself/God
lack of mercy	

What follows is a sample prayer in which one may insert a selection above for as many body parts or issues as desired. Consider also praying this over others as well as your pets.

In Jesus' name, I command and release all mountains of (insert emotion group of choice) and all mountains of trauma, shock, injury and accidents to be completely neutralized and eliminated out of wherever they are stored in my cellular programming, mind, emotional centers, spirit, and especially my (name any specific parts or areas of complaint).

I release them from all events of my life, birth, gestation, and from any iniquities or genetic imprints from my mother's and father's lineage, back through all generations. I command all evil spiritual oppressions, if present, to go from my life, family, and home.

I ask forgiveness for any sins associated with these issues (name anything that comes to mind).

I thank God for this gift and the freedom His Son has provided. If the Son has set me free; I am free indeed! I claim this as a Christian.

In the vacancies that these releases create, I accept God's love, joy, peace, patience, kindness, goodness, faithfulness, gentleness, self-control, courage, strength, forgiveness, compassion toward others, and encouragement, as well as the vibrant healthy cellular patterns as He originally intended for me to have. I give thanks in advance for all healing that God chooses to graciously grant. Amen.

Don't overdo these releases or you may feel exhausted and out of sorts, as toxins may also release. I do one emotional group once or twice weekly. To assist my body through these shifts, I mix two cups of Epsom salts mixed with 1/4 tsp lavender essential oil in a bath for 18 minutes once or twice weekly.

One may enhance the above prayer and any similar type of prayer with Appendix III. Persevere regularly until you feel the changes you desire in your body, mind, emotions, and spirit.
Just as you exercise regularly to achieve results, these may likewise require persistence until the entire stronghold is chipped away.

Appendix III

Renew Your Mind, Transform Your Body

One's thoughts are powerful and may become healthy or disease-causing blueprints within our bodies. Consider weekly meditations on a few sections below that resonate with your spirit. I release the imbalance aloud from "my entire created being" and "all cellular programming." I replace vacancies with the healthy patterns listed and add any extra pertinent issues that I choose.

WHEN THE HEAD HAS CHALLENGES
The head is especially vulnerable to negative, toxic thinking.
- I release all obsessive, self-destructive, depressive thoughts and negative focuses.
- I release any critical, unforgiving spirit toward society, others, God, or myself.
- I release all poor insight and imagination, blindness to truth, resistance to change, poor memory and attention span, addictions, distractions, obsessions, and inability to set goals for the future. I release all challenges with math, language skills, and following directions.
- I release all stored dental, hearing, and sight traumas, as well as all words I have at one time needed to say but stifled and stuffed out of fear of what others would think or say.

WHEN THE HEAD IS HEALTHY
This entwines with the intellect, thoughts, eyes, and ears.
- I live in the present. I feel totally alive and content.
- I see and hear properly. I see beauty in all creation.
- I perceive truth correctly. I am confident of God's help and wisdom.
- I love and appreciate wholesome literature and music, science and mathematics.
- I claim perfect healing of my head, ears, hearing, eyes, vision, jawbone and marrow, nerves, gums, and teeth.
- I am proficient with names and recalling details. I am intelligent and learn well.
- My mouth speaks what needs to be said--gently, courageously, and with love, always aiming to restore healthy relationships.

MAINTENANCE
- I see the good in everything.
- I have daily thankfulness, blessing those who did me wrong and returning good for evil.
- I see those who did me wrong as not my enemy but as wounded within themselves.
- I daily capture any negative thoughts and reject them.

WHEN THE THROAT HAS CHALLENGES
- I release all stuffed words as well as lack of harmony in my beliefs and what I speak.
- I release all fear of what others will think or say.
- I release all stressors from my throat, voice, thyroid, parathyroid, nerves, and cellular programming.

WHEN THE THROAT IS HEALTHY

- I feel free to speak my thoughts and feelings in a gentle, honest,and respectful manner.
- Sharing truth and knowledge with others is easy for me.
- I claim perfect healing of my throat, thyroid, parathyroid, voice, and neck.

MAINTENANCE

- I gently speak the truth with the goal of having honest and truthful relationships.
- I express myself appropriately and wisely.
- I accept that my beliefs and feelings are valid, even when in the process of meeting another's needs.
- I embrace life's changes and cycles.

WHEN THE CHEST IS CHALLENGED

- I release all forms of stored grief, sorrow, abandonment, heart wounds, loneliness, depression, hardness of heart, conflicts with men, women, children, society, God, and myself, as well as all unhealed betrayals that have ever stored in my chest, breasts, heart, lungs, breathing mechanisms, and elsewhere in my created being.
- I release poor organizational ability, lack of self-discipline, low self-esteem, emotional neediness and clinging to others, as well as unhealthy invasion of another's privacy and life.
- I let go of being excessively judgmental or excessively compassionate ("wimpy").

WHEN THE CHEST IS HEALTHY

- I easily love and trust, using wisdom in the process.
- I have courage around others, not fearing their judgments.

- I am satisfied with the love I am receiving. My God supplies all my needs.
- I cry and grieve when needed. I let go of my sorrows in a timely way and move on.
- I have a healthy balance between judgment and mercy.
- I claim perfect healing of all heart cells and energies, its valves, heartbeat mechanisms, lungs, breasts, and diaphragm.

MAINTENANCE

- I accept God's ability to heal my heart, filling it with His all-sufficient love and peace, restoring 'beauty for ashes'.
- I forgive quickly and release all injustices to God.
- I express gratefulness daily.

WHEN THE LIVER/GALLBLADDER AND SMALL/LARGE INTESTINES ARE CHALLENGED

If serious health challenge, please gain mastery over this group.

- I release all forms and all levels of stored anger, hurt, conflicts, hatred, rage, bitterness and unforgiveness. I release all irritability, depression, fear, worry, anxiety, stress, and tension.
- I release resentments and the need for revenge. I forgive all others, relatives, society, my co-workers, self, and God.
- I forgive all women and men in my life for any lack of nurture or care and for any ill-treatment or abuse.

WHEN THE LIVER/GALLBLADDER AND SMALL/LARGE INTESTINES ARE HEALTHY

- I am able to forgive myself for all my past mistakes. I forgive others easily.
- I see myself as a creation of great worth. I am organized and accomplished. I approach all obstacles with a positive outlook

and confidence.

- I allow myself to have righteous anger over injustices, but I channel it into positive action.
- I claim perfect healing over all created parts of my liver, gallbladder, small and large intestines, bowel flora, immunity, and all of their functions and nerves.

MAINTENANCE

- I regularly forgive all who wrong me—both those in the present and those from past issues that surface from time to time.
- I let go of others' imperfections, as they are a work in progress, just as I am.
- I rely on the legal system and God for justice.
- I make amends with others in person when possible or release it in private when not.
- I make restitution when possible for my wrongdoing.
- My God's love and support supplies all of my needs.
- I am a created masterpiece and beloved.

WHEN THE STOMACH IS CHALLENGED

- I release all forms and levels of worry, fear, anxiety, nervousness, stress and tension.
- I release all patterns of poor or incomplete digestion.
- I stop proclaiming: "my allergies," "I can't digest ____," and so on. Twenty times daily for as long as it takes, I proclaim, "I can perfectly digest all that I eat!"

WHEN THE STOMACH IS HEALTHY

- I have mastered spiritual peacefulness during times of stress.
- I have worked on being content in all things. I wait on the Lord's timing.

- I can accept that life contains suffering as well as happiness.
- I joyfully embrace change and new experiences knowing the Lord holds my hand. His plans for me are good.
- I claim perfect healing of all created parts and cells of my stomach, its nerves, muscles, and digestion.

MAINTENANCE
- I daily cultivate peace, tranquility, security, and trust in God.
- I make peace with the past and have hope in my future.
- I verbally express trust in God and take courage in His strength. He is my shield. I release all fears of death.
- I realize that in old age, I am closest to becoming fully alive!

WHEN THE PANCREAS IS CHALLENGED
- I release all thoughts that life is a chore and obligation.
- I release all depressions and inability to play.
- I release all resentments over growing up too soon, losing my childhood, or not having perfect parents.
- I release all workaholic tendencies. I am devoted to my family.

WHEN THE PANCREAS IS HEALTHY
- I enjoy the world's beauty. I enjoy playing and having fun.
- I claim and cultivate balance in my time spent with God, family, friends, and work.
- I claim perfect healing of all digestive, energy, and blood sugar mechanisms and their created cells and parts.
- I stop to 'smell the roses.' I balance work and play.

MAINTENANCE
- I rejoice in each new day.
- I accept joy and play daily.

- I spend time with children.
- I act maturely and responsibly.
- My God and family are a priority.
- I take time to rest.

WHEN THE ABDOMEN AND SEXUAL ORGANS ARE CHALLENGED

- I release all thoughts and feelings of being unloved, unwanted, insecure, needy, or empty.
- I release all digestive imbalances, as well as being too thin or overweight. I verbally release stored emotions from fat cells.
- I release all abuse or neglect from any individual or group.
- I release all thoughts and feelings of instability, abandonment, addiction, or uprootedness.
- I release all misuse of sex, shame, guilt, lust, and fear associated with my sexuality or fertility. I use sex properly. I release all conflicts and difficulty enjoying the opposite sex.

WHEN THE ABDOMEN AND SEXUAL ORGANS ARE HEALTHY

- I am content with my money, food, and clothing. God supplies all my needs.
- I allow God's promises and Scriptures to satisfy all the love, nurturing, stability, security, and belonging that I crave. (No human being is up for this task.)
- I enjoy and am content with the body and sexuality that God gave me. My body does not define me. It is simply my mobile home while on Earth.
- I claim perfect abdominal organs, fertility, and sexual function as was intended for me by God.

MAINTENANCE

- I place my security in God and His promises for my needs.
- I am a created, beloved masterpiece.
- I have forgiven all past wrongs or abuse.
- I enjoy my sexuality and respect the loving boundaries God has given for single and married life.

WHEN THE URINARY SYSTEM IS CHALLENGED

This also governs the bones, knees, and ears.

- I release all forms and levels of fear, worry, anxiety, terror, stress, shyness, and timidity.
- I release any lack of "backbone" and feelings of cowardice.
- I release all feelings of abandonment and instability in my life.
- I release all shock, traumas, accidents, surgeries, and combat that affects any aspect of my being.
- I release all obstacles to health in my kidneys, knees, ankles, legs, spinal cord, ears, and nerves.

WHEN THE URINARY SYSTEM IS HEALTHY

- I am building a healthy foundation for my life. I accept and trust God's care.
- I claim perfect healing of my skeleton, joints, spine, knees, spinal cord, ears, and nerves, and all their cells.
- I claim perfect kidney and urinary parts, hearing, and the ability to focus.
- I proclaim God's strength and courage when I feel weak or when adversity arises.

MAINTENANCE

- I transform all fears into courage by acting with conviction and integrity.

- I claim God as my Shield, Protector, and Refuge and realize His constant perfect love for me. People cannot truly do anything to me.
- I make peace with death and my eternity.

WHEN THE SKELETAL SYSTEM IS CHALLENGED

- I release all deep resentments, unforgiveness, hatreds, conflicts, bitterness, fear, terror, worry, anxiety, traumas, misalignments, toxins, accidents, and injuries from all of my bones, bone marrow, joints, joint fluids, all tendons and ligaments, as well as all spinal bones and disks.
- I remove my "wishbone" and grow a backbone made of action and courage.

WHEN THE SKELETAL SYSTEM IS HEALTHY

- I fill all my bones, marrow, joints, joint fluid, all tendons and ligaments, as well as my spinal bones and disks with forgiveness of all men and women, myself, and God, as well as love, joy, and courage to act on my convictions.
- I claim God's perfect patterns of healing, restoration, and alignment in all my created skeletal parts and attachments.

MAINTENANCE

- I forgive and release all offenses and related emotions before the sun goes down, if possible.
- I change my focus to the deed instead of the person. They are a work in progress and created by God.

Some of these patterns may be complex and require patience to clear—like peeling layers off of an onion. Persevere. Satan works hard at distracting us from these tasks.

I keep the Trauma Prayer in Appendix IV at hand and apply its principles also to the body parts I am addressing, especially those with difficult patterns or if pain is present. I suggest completing all the above sections at your own pace and repeating any as often as needed.

Results may take time, or you may see an immediate miracle depending on where the tipping point of the issue lies. Either way, know that a positive, healthy shift is occurring each time.

Note: some of these physical and emotional pairings are adapted from concepts in *Tools for Healing: Body, Mind and Spirit* by Steven Horne, Nature's Field 1992 — www.treelite.com as well as concepts from the book, *Chinese Constitutional Medical Model of Physical and Emotional Health: Your Nature, Your Health* by S. Dharmandanda, PhD, as well as from my long-term client biofeedback data and observations.

Body Systems and Their Parts

Some of you may wish to name additional parts of the body, specifically in trauma and emotional release. Here are the major body systems and some of their parts. I made two large posters with pictures from an anatomy booklet for my own visual reference. It has come in handy many times.

Immunity

All lymph vessels, tissues, and nodes, including the tonsils, adenoids, and appendix; the thymus gland, bone marrow, white blood cells, all energy mechanisms.

Sensory

All eye parts and visual/muscular/nerve mechanisms; cornea, iris, pupil, retina. All ear/ hearing mechanisms, external ear, middle ear, inner ear, eardrum, Eustachian tubes, auditory nerve.

Dental

All teeth, gums, tongue, jaw, marrow, TMJ joints, nerves, muscles, circulation.

Respiratory

All sinuses, trachea, lungs, bronchi, diaphragm, breathing-control centers in the brain.

Circulatory

All parts of the heart, its valves, heart beat mechanisms, nerves, arteries, veins, capillaries, and their valves, blood pressure mechanisms, the spleen, blood.

Digestion
Saliva glands, esophagus, stomach, liver, gallbladder, stomach, pancreas, small intestines, large intestines, intestinal flora, appendix, ileo-cecal valve; protein, carbohydrate, and fat digestion.

Endocrine/Hormones
Pituitary, pineal, hypothalamus, thyroid, parathyroid, adrenal glands, pancreas; blood sugar controls, weight controls, energy, and anti-aging mechanisms.

Male System
Testicles, penis, prostate, vas deferens, urethra, ureters, all sexual vitality centers, all reproductive and sexual response mechanisms.

Female System
Ovaries, fallopian tubes, uterus, cervix, vagina, external female organs, all sexual vitality, reproductive, and sexual response mechanisms.

Urinary
Kidneys, bladder, urethras, ureters, all mechanisms of mineral and fluid balance and release.

Structural System
All bones, including the skull, those in the ear, jaw, spinal column and discs, pelvis, pubic bone, tailbone, ribs, sternum; all joints—including shoulders, jaw, elbows, wrists, fingers, hips, knees, ankles, toes, tendons, ligaments, connective tissues, skin.

Nervous System
All nerves of the brain, body, spinal cord.

Brain
All parts, including centers of memory, emotion, coordination, communication, social adjustment, impulse control, breathing and digestive control, sex drive, automatic responses, skeletal movement, comprehension, sleep/wake cycles, energy, sound/smell, and emotional centers, reading comprehension, entire balance top to bottom and left to right, circulation, and nerves.

Strongholds
I have noted fascinating shifts in biofeedback by regularly commanding out toxins, in Jesus' name, "to release completely at the speed I best tolerate." Here is a list that I personally use:

- All heavy metals, including aluminum, mercury, copper, lead, cadmium, and nickel.
- All types of radiations, including that from excess sun exposure, CT scans, x-rays, cell phones, power lines, TV's computers, powertools, car and airplane travel.
- All toxic effects from vaccines, including those administered in childhood, adulthood, and inherited effects.
- All toxic viruses, mold, yeast, fungus, bacterias, parasites, worms, amoeba, food poisoning organisms, all infective organisms, chemicals, pesticides and pollutants.
- All abnormal cells, unwanted scar tissue, unwanted fat, and organ/skeletal misalignments.
- What I wish to add_____

_____

_____

_____

Appendix IV

Sample Prayers for Trauma & Healing

Dear Heavenly Father,

I speak in faith to these mountains—past physical mental, emotional, and spiritual traumas that are tormenting me at any level of my created being.

I, now, with faith in God's provisions and in Jesus' name, command all components of accidents, injuries, and events, especially involving shock, fright, pain, and terror that arose from tragic interaction with anything, such as cars, people, wars, animals, doctors, surgeries, illnesses or (_____) that disrupted any of my created parts or cellular programming at any level, including my memory, to be broken off, vaporized, and removed from my entire being in the speed I can tolerate.

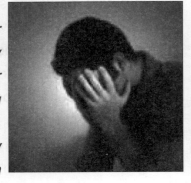

I command these removed from all events of my life, birth, gestation, and all ancestral connections that may have effected my cells, genetics, or any created parts.

The Son has set me free and I am free indeed! I claim this to fill the vacancies of all trauma patterns as well as perfect, healthy, healed patterns that God originally intended for me to have in my entire being—body, mind, emotions, and spirit. I give God glory and praise for total healing. I humbly request a creative miracle from God if needed, Amen.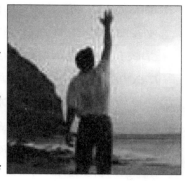

I have spoken the principle tenants of this prayer for myself, my family, and for my pets (I hold my dog and my grandchildren when I speak over them). I believe there is an element of trauma in all stored emotional pain or anytime we are blindsided physically, emotionally, and mentally. I believe some traumas take time to clear and require regular prayer and attention.

Pay special attention to current symptoms manifesting, until they are healed. As always, freely adapt this to your personal needs.

A Client's Prayer Session

This involved a young pre-teen client whose mother stated had stress from asthma. She came for biofeedback. Her mother, a Christian, gave permission to do some prayer work before we began. I offered to speak and asked if she would repeat after me. I did not record the exact prayer, but it had element of the following:

In Jesus' name, I command and release all anger, hatred, rage, bitterness, resentment, unforgiveness, sorrow, grief, heartbreak, abandonment, fear, worry, anxiety, stress, and tension of all strengths and forms to come up and out of wherever they are stored in my being, especially in my chest, heart, lungs, diaphragm, and all created breathing mechanisms. (I often have anatomy pictures to view.)

I release these from my life, birth, gestation, and from any genetic imprints and iniquities that may have come from my mother's and father's lineage back throughout all generations. I release them from any associations with others in my life and from any evil oppression that is present. I command these out during both the day and night cycles of my being. I release these emotions from all my cells, energies, nerves, thinking patterns, and spirit.

I ask forgiveness for holding onto any emotions, conflicts, or unforgiveness that should have been released. I thank God for the power within verbal speech and the freedom His Son has provided. If the Son has set me free, I am free indeed! I claim this! No weapon formed against me or my breathing mechanisms shall prosper! I can do all things through Christ who strengthens me.

I replace the vacancies this prayer creates with courage, joy, strength, peace, forgiveness, compassion toward others, love, self-control, gentleness, goodness, patience, kindness, encouragement, and perfect breathing! I command all imbalanced patterns to be replaced with vibrant healthy patterns and genetics as God originally intended, especially in my lungs, diaphragm, and breathing mechanisms.

Thank you Lord for your amazing healing provisions. Amen.

With this prayer and one session of biofeedback, her mother reported that this young lady's asthma did not reoccur when I inquired about her wellbeing a year later.

*Please be assured that I am not advocating to discard other tools of healing. Use wisdom in choosing your tools and then put as many tools into action as you feel comfortable doing. Ask God to guide you in anything else needed.

Appendix V

Godly Solutions for Healthy Sleep

In one of my classes, I was asked how one might deal with sleep challenges. I chose to search for Scriptures having to do with this topic, looking for both obstacles and aids to sleep. See if you can pick them out.

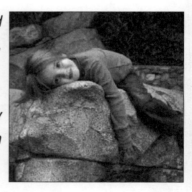

I will both lie down in peace, and sleep; for You alone, O LORD, make me dwell in safety (Ps 4:8).

Rest in the LORD, and wait patiently for Him; do not fret because of him who prospers in his way (Ps 37:7).

My son, let them not depart from your eyes--keep sound wisdom and discretion; then you will walk safely in your way, and your foot will not stumble. When you lie down, you will not be afraid; yes, you will lie down and your sleep will be sweet (Prov 3:21,23-24).

The sleep of a laboring man is sweet, whether he eats little or much; but the abundance of the rich will not permit him to sleep (Eccl 5:12).

For all his days are sorrowful, and his work burdensome; even in the night his heart takes no rest [...] (Eccl 2:23).

Now in the second year of Nebuchadnezzar's reign, Nebuchadnezzar had dreams; and his spirit was so troubled that his sleep left him. (Dan 2:1)

He shall enter into peace; they shall rest in their beds, each one walking in his uprightness (Isa 57:2).

Thus says the LORD: "Stand in the ways and see, and ask for the old paths, where the good way is, and walk in it; then you will find rest for your souls [...] (Jer 6:16).

"You said, 'Woe is me now! For the LORD has added grief to my sorrow. I fainted in my sighing, and I find no rest'" (Jer 45:3).

Come to Me, all you who labor and are heavy laden, and I will give you rest. Take My yoke upon you and learn from Me, for I am gentle and lowly in heart, and you will find rest for your souls. For My yoke is easy and My burden is light (Matt 11:28-30).

When composing the following prayers, I used my favorite basic formula: pray and command out the unwanted obstacles ('mountains'), then in their place accept and claim God's promises and gifts that reflect His Scriptural will for us.

Prayer of Release of Biblical Obstacles to Healthy Sleep

In Jesus' name, I ask forgiveness for and release all mountains of turmoil, insecurity, fear, overeating, spiritual unrest, and fretting over the riches of the wealthy. I release all sorrow, grief, pain, weariness, and all life's burdens from my mind, cells, all created sleep centers, and my entire being. I command these mountains to GO from my life, birth, gestation, and any ancestral connection and be given to the Lord to take. I am DONE with them!
(Don't stop here. Keep going to fill what emptied...)

Filling the Vacancy with Healthy Sleep Patterns

In Jesus' name, I claim peace, safety, sound wisdom, discretion, a good day's work, rest in God's care, walking uprightly on God's paths, God's protection and security to fill my body, mind, emotions, spirit, and sleep centers. I claim God's perfect patterns of rest as He intended for me to have. I thank God for His healing provisions. Amen.

Consider speaking this nightly until the transformation you desire takes place. Avoiding stimulants like caffeine and upsetting television in the evening are just a few examples of potential contributors to insomnia that you may wish to evaluate.

Appendix VI

Ellie's Prayer for the Spine

The following prayer has been adapted from Ellie, a participant in my first class who stated that she has been able to stop her dependency on other measures after regularly using this prayer. Thank You, Ellie, for sharing it. The prayer has since helped many others. We cannot claim this prayer as a substitute for your chiropractor or doctor. If you have any concerns about your spinal health, please consult your physician.

In the power of Jesus' name, I speak to my spine and command it to be loosed from all bindings.

(Speak to each area of your spine. We have been told scripturally to cultivate self-control. Use it! Pause when doing this and let the spine stretch and move around a bit—sometimes you will be aware of it shifting.

Start with number 1 and speak the *paragraph below it. Then, beginning with number 2, repeat the same *paragraph again. Do this with number 3 and 4 as well.)

I speak to:

1. My lower back, pelvis, sacrum, sacroiliac, all joints, disks, hips, and tailbone—all parts of my lower back. I also include my legs, knees, ankles, feet, and toes.
2. Middle back—including my ribs.
3. Upper back—including my collarbone, shoulders, elbows, wrists, and finger joints.
4. Neck and jaws—including my cranial bones and TMJ (jaw joints).

Be loosed from all bound-up positions. I command all my muscles, ligaments, tendons, fibers, and disks to return to their normal position, posture, strength, function, and perfect alignment in Jesus' name. I speak to all my hard tissue, soft tissue, joint fluids, and everything in between. I command all my muscles, joints and disks into position, all my vertebrae aligned, nerves unencumbered, moving freely, with perfect healing and feeling.

(Ending, after finishing with number 4):

I speak to my entire spine—anywhere that it has been compensating for any binding, misalignment, or maladjustment, and I command you to be released and loosed and returned to your normal position—to be in perfect alignment. I speak to my spine, and command it to be supernaturally and perfectly adjusted and aligned from the top of my head to the tip of my tailbone. This is all done in the name of Jesus.

Thank you, Jesus. Amen.

An Interesting Thought

The spine is encouraged to be in healthy posture when the arms are raised above the head praising the Lord.

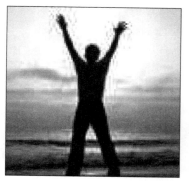

Appendix VII

Prayers for Conception & Pregnancy

A Wife's Prayer

In the name of Jesus Christ, I command and release all toxins and genetic imperfections of all strengths and sizes to come up and out of my eggs and all reproductive mechanisms now. I declare them all out from my present and past, as well as any toxic patterns passed down from my mother and father and their lineages—all the way back to Adam and Eve. I command out all negative imprints and iniquities from others, as well as any evil oppression impacting these areas. I order these out during both the day and night cycles of my being. I command these from my eggs, reproductive mechanisms, genetics, cells, energies, nerves, atoms, and molecules. In Jesus' name, I thank God—Jehovah Rapha, The Lord God Who Heals—for this gift and the freedom His Son has provided. If Christ has set me free, I am free indeed!

In the vacancies these create, I claim in Jesus' name, healthy, purified eggs, reproductive mechanisms, perfect DNA, genetic patterns, and mechanisms as God intended.

I claim perfect patterns and mechanisms for all stages of conception, all stages of fetal development, and all stages of birth to create a healthy, smart, courageous, joyful, strong, peaceful, forgiving, self-controlled, compassionate, loving, gentle, good, patient, kind, obedient, encouraging, and good-humored baby who likes to sleep at night. I replace any improper patterns at the physical, mental, emotional, and spiritual levels with vibrant healthy patterns that God intended.

Thank you, Father, for the miracle of life and for your healing provisions. Amen.

A Husband's Prayer

In the name of Jesus Christ, I command and release all toxins and genetic imperfections of all strengths and sizes to come up and out of my sperm and all reproductive mechanisms right now. I declare them all out from my present and past, as well as any toxic patterns passed down from my mother and father and their lineage—all the way back to Adam and Eve. I command out any negative imprints and iniquities from others, as well as any evil oppression impacting these areas. I order these out during both the day and night cycles of my being. I command these from my sperm, reproductive mechanisms, genetics, cells, energies, nerves, atoms, and molecules. In Jesus' name, I thank God—Jehovah Rapha, The Lord God Who Heals—for this gift and the freedom His Son has provided. If Christ has set me free, I am free indeed!

In the vacancies these create, I claim in Jesus' name, healthy, purified sperm, reproductive mechanisms, perfect

DNA, genetic patterns, and mechanisms as God intended. I claim perfect patterns and mechanisms for all stages of conception, all stages of fetal development, and all stages of birth to create a healthy, smart, courageous, joyful, strong, peaceful, forgiving, self-controlled, compassionate, loving, gentle, good, patient, kind, obedient, encouraging and good-humored baby who likes to sleep at night. I replace any improper patterns at the physical, mental, emotional, and spiritual levels with vibrant healthy patterns that God intended.

Thank you, Father, for the miracle of life and for your healing provisions. Amen.

These prayers can be adapted and applied to your children after they are born or adopted to give them a fresh start in their lives. Babies are obviously not capable of self-control or many of the other attributes listed. The prayers are intended to "plant the seed" for positive life-long characteristics that develop.

Appendix VIII

Total Forgiveness

When I Have Truly Forgiven

- I have stopped sharing with others what was done to me.
- I have made peace with others so they no longer fear me.
- I do not want them to remain in guilt. I no longer mention the issue.
- I preserve their self-esteem. I have stopped being judgmental or self-righteous.
- I let them know I will not pass on their secrets.
- I forgive aloud over and over, if needed, until I become a master of my thoughts.
- I pray for them and bless them. I give and expect nothing back.
- I no longer hold them accountable for how I am feeling.
- I believe that God forgives me. I can do no less than to forgive others. It reflects my gratefulness.
- I understand that forgiveness is a decision. I forgive the living and the dead, all men and women, society, and God (for what I mistakenly blame Him for).
- I forgive myself.
- I make restitution to others if possible to be at peace with myself and help others forgive me.

Appendix IX

Cleansing Your Home

Cleansing Your Home

- I look for any books, movies, magazines, pictures, and other objects that I feel would offend God, and I get rid of them.
- I toss out family heirlooms that would offend God.
- If good luck charms are taking the place of God, I toss them.
- If old love letters and other objects from old flames are competing for my affection towards my spouse, I clear them out.
- I look for any games and toys that have occult themes and destroy them.
- I check out my seasonal décor. If any glorifies dark forces or evil, I throw it away.
- I rid my home of any statues of gods or idols that would take my affection from God.
- I control what I watch on TV or my computer. If I struggle in this area, I will remove them from my home. They are not worth the affections of my spouse and children or any rift they create. I seek a clear conscience when I pray to my Heavenly Father.

Appendix X

Testimonies

"After having released an emotion, I usually felt calmer, had more energy and overall felt better. I also noticed my blood pressure was lower after a release of emotion or emotions."
- Ruth B.

"Using prayer to treat my long-time anxiety has been incredibly effective. I often experience instantaneous relief when I cast out fearful feelings in Jesus' name. When those feelings are a little more stubborn, I keep praying until they are gone. The Lord has never failed to deliver me when I remember to call on Him. Thanks and praise be to God."
- Alison W.

"On Sept 9, 2008, I began to develop symptoms in my throat. These symptoms were congruent with the feeling of a stuck pill or capsule in my upper throat (epiglottis). The occurrence was always unexpected and at the same intensity. It would always occur after eating foods that I have eaten many times in my life, and after it occurred with one food, it would not develop again with the same food at a later date. I have no known food allergies

and this mystery perplexed me. These symptoms occurred about every three days. After a month of using the Pearl technique (identifying parts of my neck verbally, speaking out emotions from them, and affirming the return of a healthy pattern), I no longer had such symptoms, not even in the slightest form. Glory to Jesus Christ, forever and ever!"
- Jon R.

"After a session of biofeedback working on stress patterns associated with weight and speaking out emotions for 10 minutes of that hour-long session, I lost 10 pounds."
- Trisha W.

"After having a rash on my head that was stubborn to release, I had several people verbally pray over it with me and release the "hot" emotions (anger, rage, hatred, etc.) from the skin, head, and scalp areas. The rash was gone in a week."
- Ruth H.

"I went through nine weeks of The Pearl Box study and put it into practice. Warts on my hands, which had received multiple conventional treatments over the years with no response, disappeared during the study. As I prayed off emotions of sorrow, anger, fear, and unforgiveness, my self-esteem renewed and confidence grew. My faith was strengthened as I learned to speak out God's truths for me. My immune system was fortified as a result [...] As friends and I prayed together, God also peeled off the fibromyalgia I've had a layer at a time. 13 years after its onset, I am amazed and delighted to celebrate complete healing.
- Lynn H., follow her blog at www.lynnhare.com

"As I went through the Pearl Class, I had arthritis in my hands. I felt compelled to deal with an issue of unforgiveness with my ex-husband and we talked. I shared my feelings and also verbally forgave him. My arthritis began to leave after that, and it has stayed gone ever since."
- Dale L.

"At a time where I felt a lot of fear and worry over finances and other areas of my life where I would wake up with dread and stomach pain, I began claiming for myself a truth of God: 'Jesus Christ is Lord of all,' and 'God's grace is sufficient for me.' This has since eradicated my worry. In its place has been ushered a feeling of peace that I can literally feel healing my body as I pronounce it when I awake and throughout the day."
- Bethany T.

Received via email
"In November, I went to California for my grandmother's memorial service and stayed with my aunt and uncle. I told my aunt about *The Pearl Box* class and how praying emotions out made such a big difference for each of us. My aunt had been kidnapped as a child and in the years since has lived with crippling fear and anxiety.

The morning I was to leave, I felt like I HAD to ask if I could pray with her. We did the fear prayer from the book (I brought it with me!) and then it was time for me to get on a plane. Although we are close, we do not talk or email often, but I got an email from her yesterday. She wrote that when we prayed together she felt a great heat wash over her body and knew that God was starting to heal her.

She claims Psalm 27:1-3 over herself every day and through

the Lord, is kicking fear's butt. I was so encouraged to hear that and thought you would like to hear it too.

'The Lord is my light and my salvation—whom shall I fear? The LORD is the stronghold of my life—of whom shall I be afraid? When evil men advance against me to devour my flesh, when my enemies and my foes attack me, they will stumble and fall. Though an army besiege me, my heart will not fear; though war break out against me, even then will I be confident' (Ps 27:1-3)."
- Allison W.

"I have had a life-long battle with fear that began with a mother and father that entertained and spoke fear, worry, and anxiety. This was compounded with some generational contributions by an alcoholic grandfather. My entertainment of fear kept me from stepping out of my comfort zone with the exception of occasional bouts of risk-taking.

About 17 years ago, I had an unsuccessful jaw surgery. Shortly, panic attacks became routine coupled with various physical and nervous manifestations. I coped by seeing a multitude of traditional and natural doctors. I evaluated herbal medicine, which gave me the best assistance and relief at the time, but it was not the cure. A majority of my symptoms abated about four years ago. I felt my best at that time, but then slid backward into my symptoms again.

My son's military deployment and father's death gave me awareness that some fear had been suppressed. Night terrors began. I immersed myself in the Word, prayer, counsel from godly women, and read the book, *A More Excellent Way*, by Henry Wright. When studying *The Pearl Box*, I received true clarity on the steps required to be victorious over this life-long enemy. Realizing my fears could be conquered by God's Scriptural tools truly empowered me.

Then, a second deployment order came for my son. Night terrors returned as he made plans to leave. I realized my work was not yet complete. I was so weary of this pattern and was ready for immediate change. I knew Christ's power could overcome. I enlisted friends to stop me when I was proclaiming any negative words toward myself. I decided to stop allowing my mind to feed on the news, and I memorized Scriptures to control my thoughts. I wanted to fight the fear without crutches. I wanted God to take the reins of my mind and emotions. I wrote down my thoughts, useful principles, and Scriptures the Lord gave me to live by. I used Scriptural proclamations and prayer to treat myself and rid these patterns.

I can now claim victory over this long struggle. I am currently staying alone for two weeks, which I had not been able to do before. I am sleeping soundly without any aids and without fear! It has become a whole new world for me. I have taken on new responsibilities at church. Normally, I would not have the physical and emotional strength to this. Praise God for the strength and power He has given to all of us!"

- René M.

Note: testimonies are an individual's experience and not necessarily transferrable to others. No claims are being made.

Appendix XI

The Teacup Story

A couple vacationing in Europe went strolling down a little street, and saw a quaint little gift shop with a beautiful teacup in the window. The lady collected teacups, and she wanted this one for her collection. So she went inside to buy the teacup, and as the story goes, the teacup spoke, and said:

"I want you to know that I have not always looked so lovely. It took the process of pain to bring me to this point. You see, there was a time when I was just a lump of clay and my master came and he pounded me and I screamed, "Stop that!" but he just smiled and said, "Not yet."

Then, wham! I was placed on a spinning wheel, and suddenly I was spun around and around and around. "Stop it! I'm getting dizzy! I'm going to be sick!" I screamed. But the Master only nodded and said "Not yet." He spun me, and he poked and prodded me, and he bent me out of shape to suit himself.

Then he put me in an oven, shut the door, and turned up the heat. I could see him through the oven as it was getting hotter and hotter and I thought, "He's going to burn me to death!" I never felt such heat. I yelled and knocked and pounded at the door. "Help! Get me out of here!" I could read his lips as he shook his head from side to side, "Not yet."

When I thought that I couldn't bear it another minute, the oven door opened. He carefully took me out and put me on a shelf, and I began to cool. Oh, that felt so good! "Ah, this is much better," I thought.

But after I cooled, he picked me up and he brushed and painted me all over. The fumes were horrible. I thought I would gag. "Oh, please, stop it!" I cried. He only shook his head and said, "Not yet!"

Then very gently he picked me up again and put me back into the oven. Only it was not like the first time. This time it was twice as hot, and I just knew I would suffocate. I begged. I pleaded. I screamed. I cried. I was convinced I would never make it. I could see that he was smiling, but I also noticed a tear trickle down his cheek as I watched him mouth the words, "Not yet!" I was ready to give up. Just then the door opened and he took me out, and again placed me on the shelf where I cooled. I waited and waited, wondering, "What's he going to do to me next?"

An hour later, he brought me down from the shelf. He said to me, "There, I have created what I intended. Would you like to see yourself?" He handed me a mirror and I looked, but what I saw in the mirror was so beautiful. I looked again and I said, "That's not me, I'm just a lump of clay."

He said, "Yes, that is you, but it took the process of pain to bring you to this place. You see, had I not worked you when you were clay, then you would have dried up. If I had not subjected you to the stress of the wheel, you would have crumbled. If I had not put you into the heat of the oven, there would be no color in your life. But it was the second that gave you the strength to endure. Now you are everything I intended you to be—from the beginning."

And I, the teacup, heard myself saying something I never thought I would hear myself say, "Master, forgive me. I did not trust you. I thought you were going to harm me. I did not know you had a glorious future and a hope for me. I was too shortsighted, but I want to thank you. I want to thank you for the suffering. I want to thank you for the process of pain. Here I am and I give you myself. Fill me, pour from me, use me as you see fit. I really want to be a vessel that brings you glory within my life."

The Lord knows what He's doing for each of us: He is the potter and we are His clay. He will mold us and make us, and expose us to just enough pressures of just the right kinds that we may be made into a flawless piece of work to fulfill His good, pleasing, and perfect will.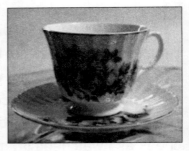

So when life seems hard, and you are being pounded and patted and pushed almost beyond endurance, when the world seems to be spinning out of control, when you feel like you are in a fiery furnace of trials, when life seems too hard to bear, try this…brew a cup of your favorite tea in your prettiest teacup; then sit down and have a little talk with the Master.

-Author Unknown

Endnotes

1. *Be in Health. It's a New Day DVD*, Henry and Donna Wright. www.beinhealth.com.

2. *What the Bible Says About Healthy Living*, Rex Russell, M.D. Ventura, CA: Regal Books. 1996.

3. *The Grape Cure*, Johanna Brandt. New York: Ehret Literature Publishing Co. (No date listed by publisher.)

4. *The Death of Cancer*. Dr. Harold Manner. Chicago, IL: Advanced Century Publishing. 1978. (I heard Dr. Manner speak on this topic, but this book is listed for further reading.)

5. Excellent quality water purification units and Pharmaceutical grade (highest quality) herbs and essential oils can be purchased at www.equippedtoheal.com.

6. *The True Power of Water*. Masaru Emoto. Hillsboro, OR: Beyond Words Publishing, Inc., 2005. pp.11-17.

7. *The Blue Zone*. Dan Buettner. Published by National Geographic Society, Washington D.C, March 2008.

8. *Aromatherapy: The Essential Beginning*. Gary Young. Salt Lake City, Utah, Essential Press Publishing, 1996. p.39. pp.132-153 give an alphabetical list of single essential oils and their common and historical usages.

9. *What They Don't Want You to Know About the Healthcare System*. Sound Concepts, Inc., 2008. Brochures can be ordered at www.naturestools.com or www.ReadingIsLeading.com.

10. International Standard Bible Encyclopaedia, Electronic Database Copyright 1996 by Biblesoft

11. I was privileged to hear Dr. John Christopher speak in person at the National Health Federation conventions during the 1970s in Portland, Oregon.

12. *Change Your Brain, Change Your Life*. Dr. Daniel Amen M.D. (PBS special, 2008).

13. *Horsefeathers* CD, Dr. Carl Hammerschlag, M.D. This can be purchased at www.healingdoc.com. (I especially appreciated Hammerschlag's urging to re-examine our old belief systems.)

14. *Change Your Brain, Change Your Life*. Dr. Daniel Amen M.D. PBS special, 2008.

15. *The Work*, Byron Katie Mitchell. Used with written permission. See "Loving What Is" on her website, www.thework.com

16. *The Significance of Saying*. Keith Moore. Moore Life Ministries, Branson, MO. Audio Tapes 2002.

17. *Tools for Healing: Body, Mind and Spirit Student Workbook,* Steven Horne. Utah, Nature's Field, 1992. This tool includes the concept of what he called the "voodoo hex," as well as cultural concepts of specific emotions associated with specific organs or systems. His website is www.treelite.com, where one may access Tree of Light Publishing.

18. *Love, Medicine, and Miracles.* Bernie Siegel. Quill Publishing, 1986.

19. *The Significance of Saying.* Keith Moore. Moore Life Ministries, Branson, MO. Audio Tapes 2002.

20. Ibid.

21. *Managing Your Mood.* Steven Horne. Nature's Sunshine Convention Seminar. Washington. D.C. 2008. (He provided a great framework to separate and categorize emotional groupings.)

22. *Your Nature, Your Health.* S. Dharmananda. Portland, OR, Institute for Traditional Medicine and Preventative Health Care. 1986. pp.35,36, 216-236. (I took his class years ago and reviewed general concepts related to physical/emotional connections that are congruent with Chinese medicine. I then included common physical/emotional relationships from my clinical work and biofeedback sessions using concepts of Chinese medicine that I have utilized throughout the past 20 years, including a visit to China where I reviewed Chinese Constitutional Medicine in Beijing.)

23. *A More Excellent Way.* Pastor Henry Wright. Molena, GA,

Pleasant Valley Church, Inc., 1999. pp.128, 171-173, 209, 236.

24. *Facing the Giants* DVD. Destination Film. 2006.

25. Art Matthias. www.akwellspring.com.

Additional tools for group Bible study

- Don Colbert, *The Seven Pillars of Health*. www. sevenpillarsofhealth.com. This is a great DVD set for use while studying the pearls of physical health.
- Henry and Donna Wright. www.beinhealth.com. This website gives more tools for advanced study on the spiritual roots of disease. I utilize the DVD series, *A New Day*, in my classes.
- YouTube: Paul Nisan. Lecture excerpts from his book, *Health According to the Scriptures*. Some of what he has to say is quite thought provoking.
- moorelifeministries.org. God's Will to Heal CD's. Keith Moore has a lot of free material that he makes available.
- Life Outreach International, *Your Body, His Temple* DVD series. www.lifetoday.org.

Four of my favorite tools for physical health

THE ZYTO COMPASS

This is a relatively inexpensive device that tests the body with cutting edge technology in about five minutes using your right hand. It analyzes imbalanced body parameters and matches the client with excellent precision to the supplements they need. No more guessing! This is a fabulous tool for health practitioners, but is also worthwhile for families.

QUALITY SUPPLEMENTS

We recommend and distribute the Nature's Sunshine Products line of quality herbs, extracts, liquid tonics, and essential oils harvested from carefully chosen raw materials all over the world. Nature's Sunshine is all about purity and potency. Their products are certified GMP (Good Manufacturing Practices) and Pharmaceutical Grade, which is a grade beyond organic.

THE NRG FOOTBATH

We also love the NRG footbath machine to assist the entire body in its health journey. We love how the NRG Footbath gives the body energy as a tool for healing. Many have felt that it has accelerated their healing process. We have personally found it to be supportive of the natural detoxification process of the body.

THE ORIGINAL RICHWAY AMETHYST BIO-MAT

This is a mat releasing healing far-infrared waves enhanced by quality amethyst to provide energy, pain relief, and more to the body. I provide these for clients and educate them thoroughly as to their use. Its impact on the circulatory, skeletal, digestive, and immune system is extraordinary. All therapies including nutritional seem to work better with this. I wish everyone owned one. All one does is lie or sleep on it. It is used as a major therapy for serious health challenges in Japan.

More information and ordering options for all of the above healing tools can be obtained at: www.equippedtoheal.com